Disorders of Human Communication 1

Edited by G.E. Arnold, F. Winckel, B.D. Wyke

E. D. Schubert
Hearing: Its Function
and Dysfunction

Springer-Verlag Wien GmbH

Prof. Earl D. Schubert

Stanford Medical Center
Stanford, California, U.S.A.

Originally published by Springer-Verlag/Wien in 1980
Softcover reprint of the hardcover 1st edition 1980

With 86 Figures

Library of Congress Cataloging in Publication Data. Schubert, Earl D. 1916—. Hearing, its function
and dysfunction. (Disorders of human communication ; 1.) Bibliography: p. Includes index. 1. Hearing
disorders. 2. Hearing. 3. Psychoacoustics. I. Title. II. Series. [DNLM: 1. Ear-Physiology. 2. Hearing
disorders. 3. Hearing. W1 DI762 v. 1 / WV270 S384h.] RF290.S4. 617.8'86. 80-23338

ISBN 978-3-7091-3363-7   ISBN 978-3-7091-3361-3 (eBook)
DOI 10.1007/978-3-7091-3361-3

Editors' Foreword

This volume is one in a series of monographs being issued under the general title of "Disorders of Human Communication". Each monograph deals in detail with a particular aspect of vocal communication and its disorders, and is written by internationally distinguished experts. Therefore, the series will provide an authoritative source of up-to-date scientific and clinical information relating to the whole field of normal and abnormal speech communication, and as such will succeed the earlier monumental work "Handbuch der Stimm- und Sprachheilkunde" by R. Luchsinger and G. E. Arnold (last issued in 1970). This series will prove invaluable for clinicians, teachers and research workers in phoniatrics and logopaedics, phonetics and linguistics, speech pathology, otolaryngology, neurology and neurosurgery, psychology and psychiatry, paediatrics and audiology. Several of the monographs will also be useful to voice and singing teachers, and to their pupils.

August 1980

G. E. Arnold, Jackson, Miss.
F. Winckel, Berlin
B. D. Wyke, London

Preface

Despite years of interest and research in the hearing process, much of the exact detail of auditory processing remains in the realm of conjecture. We *do* have some rudimentary understanding of the way the system records changes in frequency and intensity and of the relations between the ear's spectrum analysis and our identification of sound quality. Some of these operations we can duplicate with auditory models of our own, or with laboratory analyzers that can serve as auditory analogs. But the complex, rapidly-changing signals that constitute speech, for example, are processed with a very low error rate by the normally-operating auditory system; and this is accomplished even in the presence of interference or distortion that would render our other sophisticated analyzing systems virtually useless.

This low ceiling on our comprehension of the system is distressing, but fortunately it does not greatly diminish the interest in the auditory process of many experts in fields related to hearing. It is primarily for this group of interested scholars that this book has been written—specifically those with expertise in a related field such as medicine, psychology, physics, engineering, etc. For this reason an effort has been made to keep the treatise brief enough to avoid burdening the interested outsider with more than he wishes or needs to know about hearing. In the same vein, very little time is spent on historical background. For the student who intends to make hearing itself his specialty, this work provides a highly useful overview and many convenient signposts directing the reader to supplementary information.

With this same group of experts in mind, it is not necessary to repeat the basic technical background information required for understanding what we currently can explain of the operation of the auditory system. The beginning audiologist, for example, might find it necessary to fill elsewhere his need for some grounding in elementary principles of sound transmission, basic physiology and neurophysiology, and experimental psychology in order for the material as presented here to be sufficiently comprehensible.

Several topics, among them the role of the auditory system in the perception of music, and the principles of the processing of speech are quite fully covered in other volumes of this same series, but they come in for some attention here because such integrated responses definitely influence our analysis of certain specific auditory dimensions or operations.

For a fairly cohesive overview of the hearing process, reading the chapters in order is the recommended procedure. For a reader whose immediate interest is in a specific aspect, the separate chapters are reasonably independent and contain sufficient references to be of additional guidance.

Not much space is given to auditory theory, since what theories we do have encompass very narrow aspects of auditory operation and fall woefully short of accounting for anything save the most elementary aspects of auditory processing. In contemplating the everyday usefulness of the auditory system as a sense organ we have no theory comprehensive enough to be worth the telling. This is intended not so much as a comment on our shortcomings as scholars in audition but rather as a recognition of the complexity and versatility of the system.

In acknowledging contributions to a treatise of this sort, it's difficult to be appropriately comprehensive. Intellectually, my debt is to a great many of my fellow students of the auditory system—those whose writings and discussions have fashioned our mutual understanding of the total hearing process. Some are cited herein, but of course many are more indirectly represented. Finally, in the technical aspects of turning a manuscript into a book, I am most beholden to my willing and able spouse who took over all concerns about proper organization and form, and made certain I could concentrate on the task of writing.

Stanford, Calif., August 1980   **Earl D. Schubert**

Contents

Introduction 1

Part I. Anatomy and Physiology of the Auditory System . . . 5

1. Outer Ear 7
2. Middle Ear 11
   Middle Ear Muscles 15
3. Inner Ear 17
   Electric Potential in the Cochlea 23
   Cochlear Innervation 25
4. Frequency Analysis in the Cochlea 27
5. Central Auditory System 33

Part II. Psychoacoustics 39

6. Auditory Sensitivity 43
   Minimum Audible Pressure 45
   Minimum Audible Field 45
   Response Curve of the Ear 47
7. Frequency Analysis: Pitch 50
   The Nature of Pitch 51
   Pitch Change 53
   Simultaneous Pitches 58
   Pitch of Complex Tones 60
8. Loudness 67
9. Temporal Patterns 74
   Fusion of Signals 82
10. Spectrum Analysis 85
    Sound Quality 85
    Simultaneous Masking 91
    Auditory Filters — Critical Bandwidths 93
    Shape of the Auditory Filter 97

11. Binaural Hearing 100
    Localization of Sound 100
    Interaural Time-Pattern Analysis 108
    Signal Selection by the Binaural System 111

Part III. Hearing Loss 117

12. Conductive Loss 121
    Normal Hearing Standards 121
    Tests for Conductive Loss—The Audiogram 123
    Tympanometry 127
13. Cochlear Dysfunction 134
    Békésy Audiograms 135
    Other Cochlear Tests 139
14. VIIIth Nerve Problems 145
15. Threshold Shift 148
16. Evoked Response Audiometry 155
    Cochleography 155
    Vertex Electric Response 157
17. Central Dysfunction 161
    Tests with Speech Materials 162
18. Hearing Aids 165
19. Auditory Implants 170

References 174

Subject Index 181

Introduction

There can be little doubt that a highly diversified auditory system is a primary factor in the development of the species. The complexity of audible communication is perhaps the most discernible way in which humans excel over other animals, spoken language being possibly the most useful accomplishment in the evolution of modern man. Through the auditory channel we also receive a great deal of information about relevant happenings in the environment, but whether the human system is more versatile than other forms in interpreting non-speech sound is not so easily verified.

When we add the sounds of music to our perceptual repertoire, it seems almost self evident that the human auditory system processes a wider variety of signals than any other. Musical sounds are an especially interesting class of auditory signals, since it is difficult to find a close analog in the environment. There are few, if any, naturally occurring sequences of sound that are inherently esthetically pleasing. In vision, the artist finds scenes and patterns in nature that may be almost universally recognized as intrinsically pleasing or beautiful. In audition, pleasure from sound patterns or sequences springs almost entirely from artificially-fabricated sequences. And even though the sequences and the structure of tones may differ widely in different cultures, the existence of some pleasurable auditory ensemble seems to be universal, as does also the existence of a spoken language. So complete is our preoccupation with speech and music that by far the greater involvement with sound, at least in the modern world, centers on perception of sounds which man produces rather than on other useful sounds from the environment. How much this has influenced the evolutionary development of the human auditory system is a fascinating but presently imponderable question.

Interest in the mechanical operation of the ear is nearly as old as recorded history; but as one might expect, it originally had to do with only the visible component of the system. The external ear, according to an Egyptian papyrus dated around 1500 B.C., is the organ of hearing and also has some function related to respiration. One supposes this might be occasioned by noting the sensation of pressure equalization through the Eustachian tube.

The auditory nerve seems to have been located next, long before recognition of the middle ear and inner ear. Such a situation was not conducive to meaningful analysis of mechanical auditory function. Pythagoras, who noted that numerical simplicity of tonal ratios corresponded to heightened blend in the resulting auditory sensation had no knowledge of the anatomy of the cochlea. Nearly two centuries later Aristotle promulgated the idea of the "aer internus", the pocket of internal air behind the eardrum that was supposedly responsible for reproducing the external condition inside the body where it could be read by the internal mechanism responsible for auditory sensations.

Largely because of strictures against anatomical research by the prevailing religions, this doctrine was not challenged until the 16th century. It was still the explanation given in Koyter's book on the ear published near the close of that century. But Vesalius showed two of the small middle-ear bones in his textbook on anatomy, though not in their normal position; and late in the 17th century the form of the inner ear was quite clearly shown in DuVerney's treatise on the ear.

By the time of Helmholtz, great strides had been made and the major anatomy of the inner ear was nearly completely known; the conduction of sound in air, liquid and solids had been established, and the relation of vibrating frequency to perceived pitch had been pointed out by Galileo. Helmholtz put much of this knowledge together in formulating his hypothesis that the auditory system responded differently to different frequencies because the ear itself contained a series of tuned elements (resonators), each of them connected to a different nerve or set of nerves.

This was not the first of the resonance theories; the resonance mechanism had been invoked to explain how sound from the outside could be sensed by the brain as early as 1605 by Bauhin. Later DuVerney employed the principle to account for the separation of high and low frequencies by the ear. These are the simplest forms of the "place" theory of hearing—that the pitch of a tone is dictated by the place of stimulation, or by implication the place of origin of the responding fibers. Some interesting arguments ensued about the specific elements that could resonate suitably, and our later discussion of the structure of the inner ear will make it clear that argument could easily arise. Yet Helmholtz structured for the time a rather elegant theory. It involved an extension of Müller's doctrine of specific energy of nerves. Müller's original exposition stated that the kind of sensation experienced was determined by the particular nerve that was stimulated. Helmholtz' formulation by implication, called for different fibers of the same nerve to elicit different pitches. It also invoked the recently-formulated Ohm's law of acoustics—that the ear analyzes a complex periodic waveform into its constituent sinusoidal components.

Helmholtz' theory was accepted at first, but then became the point of departure for a host of competing theories. As is usual in the absence of direct observation or measurement, explanations proliferated and argument flourished. Békésy's direct observation of the cochlea in action sounded the death knell for many of the mechanical hypotheses, and truly ushered in the modern era of auditory research.

During the period of Helmholtz' contribution, the study of hearing was accelerated and expanded also by rising interest in the study of psychophysics—the relation between the physical stimulus to the sense organs and the resulting sensation or perception. Particularly in Germany during this period, and later in America, experimental psychologists were engaged in systematic study of responses to visual and auditory signals in the environment. Especially in audition, the advent of electronic instruments and the parallel interests of telephone engineers had a highly beneficial effect.

Our current state of understanding of the very complex operation of the auditory system is the result of individual and cooperative effort by physicians, psychologists, physiologists, engineers and audiologists. The complexities of the human visual and auditory systems are such as to tax the explanatory capabilities of the scholars who essay to understand them. So far each new discovery seems to elevate the level of description required rather than bring us closer to complete explanation. The present treatise, therefore, is destined to leave the reader with the impression that we understand the system as a complete sensory system only at a very superficial level. We know disturbingly little of the actual nature of the processing of speech or music by the system. We cannot explain how it comes about that it separates simultaneous signals far better than our own laboratory devices or computer programs, or how it operates so comparatively well in reverberant noisy environments. Perhaps the most heuristic view of this state of affairs is that it is consequently even more imperative that we continue to view what presumably *has* been established with proper skepticism, and where necessary entertain more than one tenable view of those areas that are still poorly verifiable.

This is the only attitude that seems defensible to the writer, and it is urged upon the reader throughout the remainder of this book.

Part I
Anatomy and Physiology of the Auditory System

Outer Ear 1

A highly schematized view of the parts of the peripheral auditory system is shown in Fig. 1. It is drawn for clarity rather than accuracy, and serves, for our present purposes, to highlight the relation between the outer ear and the eardrum. For reasons touched on in the introduction, the external ear has been a subject of interest longer than the rest of the system.

One of the questions seriously discussed about the time of Aristotle was "Why are man's ears stationary?" We may decide to revive this question when we discuss localization of sound. A more easily answered common-sense question about the external ear would be "Why is the eardrum so well hidden from the acoustic environment?" The easiest answer is that it needs protection and it needs to stay in calibration. And as nearly as we can tell, it suffers little or no acoustic handicap from being hidden for these physiological reasons.

The size and shape of the external and middle ear appear to be related to the wavelength of the sounds that are useful to the organism. Regarding the specific size and composition of the outer ear structures, Fig. 2 should be useful. The auricle (pinna) itself is roughly oval in shape with the longer axis about 6.5 cm and the shorter one about 3.5 cm. On the front edge of this oval is a depression known as the concha, crudely of the shape of a truncated hemisphere with a diameter of about 2.5 cm and a radius of about 1.25 cm. The ear canal sits at the front edge of the concha and is itself somewhat oval in shape at the entrance, with a height of about 0.9 cm and a width of about 0.65 cm. The canal is nearly 3.0 cm in length, with the wall of the first one-third of the length being cartilaginous and covered loosely with skin, whereas the innermost two thirds has a bony wall and a more tightly-fitting skin. At the termination of this canal is the eardrum or tympanic membrane. This is the boundary between the outer and the middle ear. It has a rather complicated shape, but loosely resembles a flat cone with an angle of about 135°, not too different from that of many loudspeaker diaphragms. Furthermore, the membrane sits at an angle in the end of the canal, so that it presents a larger

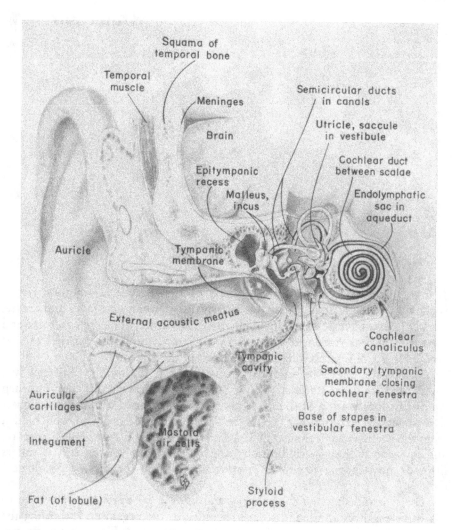

Fig. 1. Cross-section drawing of outer, middle, and inner ear of man. (From Anson and Donaldson, 1967)

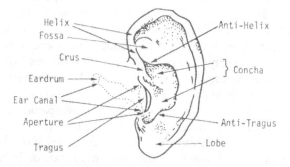

Fig. 2. The shape of the external ear and the names of its principal parts

surface to the air of the canal than it would were it normal to the axis of the canal.

Thus, so far as we have followed it, the outer ear resembles a tapering channel without too many abrupt changes that would cause reflections of the varying pressures that bring about the motions of the eardrum. In the process, the structure of the outer ear also furnishes protection for the eardrum, which, although it is a rather tough, resilient structure, would be much more subject to injury and to spurious loading by foreign material if it were located on the surface of the skull. Further special protection is afforded by the fact the canal contains a few hairs and that it has provision for secreting a wax with an apparently unpleasant effect on curious insects.

As Shaw (1974) has pointed out, these structures make very little difference to the transmission of sounds of low frequency but they do enhance the transmission of frequencies above about 1 kHz. This is shown in some detail in Fig. 3 which gives the ratio of sound pressure measured at a point outside the pinna to sound pressure at the eardrum (left ordinate) for various frequencies. It is apparent that at a 45° azimuth frequencies between 2 kHz and 5 kHz benefit considerably from the size, shape and placement of the outer ear. For sounds from other angles, the picture changes systematically, but for sounds from the front the situation is essentially the same as shown in the figure.

The outer ear, or pinna, in man functions most efficiently in the frequency range important for differentiating the sounds of speech. Whether the specific convolutions of the pinna also perform a special function in the localization of sounds has been a matter of interesting conjecture and will be discussed in

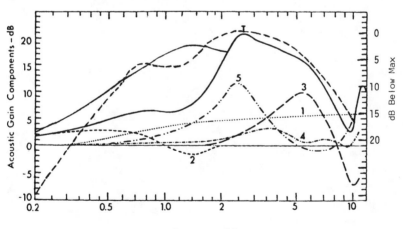

Frequency – kHz

Fig. 3. Acoustic gain contributed by each of these five components: *1* The head, assuming it is a sphere, *2* The torso and neck, *3* The concha, *4* The pinna flange, *5* The canal and eardrum. The solid curve marked T is the total gain in pressure from free field to eardrum for a source at 45° azimuth. The unnumbered dashed line represents the shape of the response of the ear at threshold. This could properly be called the sensitivity curve of the ear. Sensitivity relative to peak is shown on the right-hand ordinate. The uppermost solid curve shows the low-frequency transfer characteristic of the middle ear.
(Modified from Shaw, 1974)

a later chapter. For our present purposes it is only the gross shape that has any significance. Along with the ear canal, the pinna functions in a minor way as a smaller version of the pre-hearing-aid ear trumpet. This is part of the overall gain in sensitivity that accrues from the fact that the closed-tube resonance of the canal and the gain from the baffle effect of the concha lie in the same general frequency region. The advantage afforded by the concha begins to be effective at about the frequency region where the middle ear transfer function shows a drop in gain, namely about 1500 Hz (Møller, 1963). The concha contributes a sound pressure gain of nearly 3 to 1 in the range from 4—5 kHz (Shaw, 1974).

For additional perspective the two higher curves have been included. The solid curve shows the shape of the middle ear transfer function, and one gets a rough idea how the total curve showing the combination of the middle ear, the canal and the outer ear structures adds to the middle ear response to form the total frequency response curve of the ear as portrayed by the dotted upper curve. This is the inverse of the sensitivity or "threshold" curve of the ear, which we will later study in greater detail.

The extent to which the presence of the pinna aids in the location of sound sources has been explored only recently. This will be looked at more closely when we discuss localization of sound.

Middle Ear 2

Although the boundary is an arbitrary one, the tympanic membrane can well be considered to separate the outer from the middle ear as shown back in Fig. 1. For one thing, it is useful to consider that the action changes at that point from acoustical to mechanical, just as at a loudspeaker it changes from mechanical to acoustical. The eardrum does indeed roughly resemble the cone of a loudspeaker in shape as well as in function. Its task is to make efficient use of the sound energy from the air in driving a mechanical system, just as the properly designed mechanical loudspeaker diaphragm will efficiently *radiate* acoustic energy.

The comparison can be carried further. The center of the eardrum is quite rigid for a physiological membrane, and it is loosely mounted at the rim, especially so at the lower edge, where the pars flaccida nearly constitutes a fold in the unstressed drum.

As Davis has pointed out, the application of the term drum is most descriptive for the entire middle ear, with the tympanic membrane as the drum head. In current usage, however, eardrum is routinely taken to mean the tympanic membrane. As seen in Fig. 4, displacements of the drum resulting from changes in pressure are transmitted to the inner ear via a chain of three bones, the malleus, incus and stapes. These are suspended in the middle ear cavity as suggested by Fig. 5, and serve as a rather special transmission chain for carrying the vibrations of the drum to the fluids of the inner ear.

Actually, to understand the mechanical function of the drum and the ossicular chain one needs to consider their close coupling to the fluids of the inner ear and through the fluids to the round window pressure-release mechanism. As we shall see in the next section, it is the movement of the hairs of the hair cells by the inner-ear fluid that initiates the neural activity basic to the hearing sensation. In addition, as is apparent from consideration of Fig. 4, the air cavity of the middle ear has its mechanical effect. Its basic form mechanically is an air-filled cavity of about 1.5 cc volume with a movable diaphragm (the drum) about 0.6 cm² in area. Such a piston-driven cavity acts like a mechanical stiffness element (analogous to a spring), and its impedance

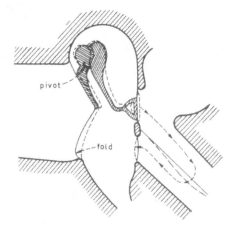

Fig. 4. Two-dimensional scheme showing the action of the middle ear. A moment of condensation (positive pressure) in the air of the ear canal forces the eardrum inward, and the structures move from the solid to the dotted position. The movement is greatly exaggerated, since the drum, which is about 0.1 mm thick moves about 1 micron or 1/100 of its thickness even for a very strong sound. Because of the way it is suspended by muscles and ligaments (not shown) the ossicular chain pivots around a point very close to its center of gravity. Note that since the eardrum and the round window membrane both move simultaneously toward the middle ear cavity the air of the middle ear cavity must be compressed during this phase of the cycle. (From Stevens and Davis, 1938)

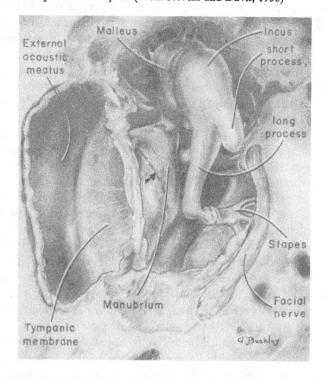

Fig. 5. Photograph of the middle ear. The canal and the middle-ear wall have been cut away to show the position of the drum, ossicles and suspending ligaments. (From Anson and Donaldson, 1967)

to a driving oscillating force doubles for every halving of the driving frequency. The effect of the presence of this middle-ear cavity, then, is to decrease the low-frequency amplitude response of the middle ear.

Over all, then, the task of the middle ear is to transfer the energy represented by the air vibration in the canal to the sensory cells of the inner ear. Converting the motion of lighter air particles into movement of the heavier liquids and tissues of the inner ear calls for the trading of greater displacement for greater force—an impedance-matching transformation. It does this rather well at low frequencies, so that in general, the effect of the drum, the middle ear cavity and the ossicular chain is to transmit frequencies below 1400 Hz with about equal displacement amplitude (this will be a velocity increase of 2 for each octave increase in frequency), but to pass frequencies above that progressively more poorly—decreasing by a factor of 4 for each octave to about 4000 Hz, where the drum ceases to behave as a single rigidly-coupled vibrator and its behavior is more erratic.

Regarding the construction of the ossicular chain, the malleus handle lies along the vertical axis of the oval-shaped drum and is firmly attached to it. The massive portion, or head of the malleus, articulates firmly with the incus and the incus in turn with the projection, or crus, of the stapes. The axis of rotation of this transmitting chain is—very nearly, at least—around its own center of gravity, thus it is readily driven (Kirikae, 1960).

Over the low-frequency range, where it works well, the middle ear may accomplish its task of lessening the impedance mismatch between the air of the canal and the structures of the inner ear by three possible complementary mechanisms. First we need to note that the concept of the rigid cone (the ear drum) driving the lever system of the ossicular chain, as intimated by the analogy to the loudspeaker or microphone, is not quite accurate. From holographic measurements of the vibration pattern of the drum, Tonndorf and Khanna (1972) noted that part of the drum moves with considerably greater amplitude than the attached malleus handle. For a time they were disposed to revive the old Helmholtz hypothesis that the ear drum adduces some mechanical advantage from operating as a curved membrane, as shown in Fig. 6. It would indeed be fascinating if the construction of the drum itself did contribute to the mechanical gain of the system. The relative amplitudes from a cross section of the drum *do* show the appropriate pattern, as in Fig. 6 B. But the drum is best viewed mechanically as an acoustically driven shell, and apparently these areas where the amplitude of the drum is greater than that of the malleus handle simply indicate that because of non-acoustic biological design restrictions it is not an ideally stiff cone. Thus greater vibration of the less-directly-attached parts of the drum probably means a loss of some of the impinging energy. With our present knowledge of the details of drum operation, this first possible mechanism of mechanical gain must be held in abeyance.

The second principle embodied in the efficient energy transfer from air through the middle ear to the inner ear is probably popularly recognized as the analog of the prybar, where the greater displacement of a longer lever arm is traded for the greater force of a shorter one. It is shown in simple form in Fig. 6 C. The more precise description is that if the force on the longer arm is

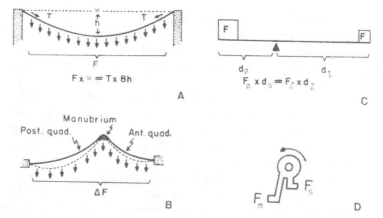

Fig. 6. Principles of the middle-ear mechanical advantage. *A* shows an idealized form of the membrane. See the discussion in the text. Whether the principle actually applies or whether the drum really behaves mechanically like a shell rather than a membrane is still controversial. *B* shows a cross section through the tympanic membrane indicating how the force is transferred to the manubrium (handle) of the malleus at one typical cross section of the drum. *C* shows the general fulcrum form of force gain; and *D* the geometric form embodied in the middle ear. (From Tonndorf and Khanna, 1970)

designated by F_l and that on the shorter by F_s, then using similar designations for the longer and shorter distances

$$F_s = (d_l/d_s)\, F_l$$

and the gain in force for the shorter lever arm is seen to be the ratio of the longer arm to the shorter. The not-quite-so-obvious form of the same principle more closely resembling the configuration in the middle ear is shown in D of Fig. 6. In this instance, the long arm is the manubrium of the malleus and the shorter one the long process of the incus. It is not really visually apparent in Fig. 5, but the pivot point of the ossicular chain is so located that the lever arm on the drum side is slightly longer than that on the stapes side of the pivot; thus some trading of greater drum displacement for greater force on stapes takes place.

Finally, and most important, the area of the tympanic membrane exposed to the vibrations of the air is considerably greater than the area of the footplate of the stapes driving the fluid of the inner ear. This acts in the same direction as the lever-arm advantage because the force on the stapes is the product of the sound pressure in the canal and the area of the drum, whereas without the drum it would be the much smaller stapes area multiplied by the pressure in the canal or the middle ear cavity. Stripped of unnecessary complications, the system looks like the portrayal in Fig. 7. The advantage gained is the ratio of the two areas.

On a superficial look, it appears that sound transmission would suffer very little if the middle ear mechanism were like the system in Fig. 7. The three-bone ossicular chain developed during the evolution of mammals, and probably served other purposes than the enhancement of sensitivity. It may offer some protection by affording a limit on amplitude displacement, but this has never been convincingly demonstrated.

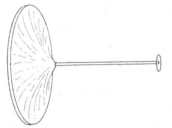

Fig. 7. Mechanical advantage afforded by drum-to-stapes area ratio. The force exerted on the small area at the right (pressing on the cochlear fluid) will be increased because of the larger area of the surface at the left (acted upon by the air in the ear canal)

None of these three complementary mechanisms for the advantageous transfer of energy through the middle ear is easy to measure precisely. Possibly the best estimates emerge from the Tonndorf and Khanna holographic measurements of eardrum vibration. Their measurements on cats are more detailed and probably represent good estimates for the middle ear of human ears. They estimated the advantage of the curved membrane as 2.0, the ossicular chain lever ratio as 1.4 and the area ratio as 34.6. Multiplying these gives a total estimated ratio gain of close to 100, meaning that the system loses 40 dB of sensitivity without the middle ear—an estimate roughly confirmed by measurement.

Thus a rather specialized device has been required if the comparatively small amount of the already small energy of sound-wave vibration in the air is to vibrate the structures of the inner ear. We have seen that the outer ear is of some help since it takes advantage of the baffle effect of the head and the pinna and adds to that the resonance effect of the ear canal. The middle ear preserves this advantage rather admirably over the low frequency range and helps to broaden the sensitivity curve of the system, as we shall see in a later discussion.

Middle Ear Muscles

In the normal ear, when the sound stimulus reaches about 75—80 dB above threshold the middle ear muscles contract and reduce the transmission efficiency of low frequency sounds. Most of this reduction appears attributable to the stapedius muscle which acts somewhat independently of the tensor tympani, the innervation of the two being different. These two small muscles can be just barely seen in Fig. 5. Just behind the long process of the incus, the tensor tympani muscle is visible, running from the manubrium of the malleus to the innerwall of the middle ear cavity. It stresses the tympanic membrane (drum) by drawing it inward. The stapedius muscle cannot be seen, but the tendon which attaches the muscle to the head of the stapes is clearly visible as it emerges from behind the facial nerve (or in front, since we are looking in from the posterior). This muscle pulls the anterior border of the footplate outward. It has been difficult to establish just what aspect of the signal acts to govern the behavior of the muscles, *i.e.*, whether it be peak excursion, energy integrated over some period, spectral composition, or possibly some less easily defined perceptual aspect such as loudness. This latter seems possible both from the nature of the response and from the fact that the reflex arc is not a simple one. (See Møller, 1974, for a synopsis.)

As a matter of fact, it seems quite unlikely that the whole middle-ear muscle complement evolved for the purpose of protection from loud sounds (Simmons, 1964). The complex innervation and the low likelihood of high-level acoustic disturbances point toward a different explanation for the evolution of such a device. Considering the nature of the suspension of the ossicles as seen in Fig. 5 and the extremely small displacements required to create very loud sounds, a more defensible explanation is that its usefulness is (or was) greater in animals in closer contact with the earth. Even in the human, the muscles are activated at times of, or prior to, movement of related structures, as during the jaw movements accompanying speech. Chances are that that proliferating breed, the American jogger, must remember to maintain a certain muscle tone to keep from hearing the small movements of his suspended ossicular chain.

By far the most interesting auditory task of the muscles, however, is their protective function. Certain aspects of this are useful in assessing hearing loss and will be discussed in later chapters.

Inner Ear   3

Of course, the truly impressive part of the pre-neural auditory system is the inner ear. Even with modern accomplishments in micro-packaging, it is doubtful that the cochlea is rivalled for the amount of processing that takes place in a given small space.

In form, the inner ear has the shape of the shell of a snail, hence the name, cochlea. A good idea of its geometric form can be gained from Fig. 1. It is wise, however, in looking at drawings of the inner ear to be constantly reminded that the structures involved are very small. The tubelike part of the cochlear passage is only about 2 mm in diameter, and since it is roughly 35 mm long, it is a much longer, narrower tube than the diagram makes it appear to be. Though there have been occasional reminders from students of its exact operation that the coiled aspect may have at least a small effect on the mechanical response of the inner ear, its detailed operation is most easily described by considering it to be straight rather than spiral. When we do adopt the simplification of straightening and shortening the cochlea for the sake of easier visualization, it can be likened roughly to the diagram in Fig. 8. Note that the basilar membrane, which is taken to be the primary mechanical element in the cochlear duct tapers in the opposite direction to the taper of the cochlea itself, being narrower at the basal end than at the helicotrema. Here, also, a diagram like Fig. 8, cannot give a true perspective, since the membrane is about. 1 mm wide at the basal end, about 0.5 mm wide at the helicotrema and is about 32 mm long. It is therefore a much longer narrower ribbon than is implied by the simplified drawing.

Looking ahead at the diagram in Fig. 10, we lose entirely our impression of the 3-dimensional configuration of the device, but it does serve to identify a number of the structures involved in its operation. To keep size in perspective, it is wise to keep in mind that in man, the scala vestibuli averages about 1 mm^2 in cross sectional area, the scala tympani roughly the same and the cochlear duct (scala media) only about one quarter mm^2. We have just noted the basilar membrane varies in width by a factor of about 5 to 1. In arriving at even a

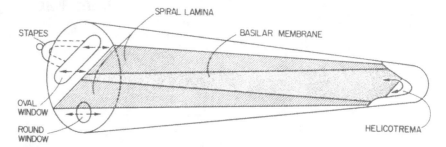

Fig. 8. Idealized uncoiled diagram of the cochlea emphasizing the controlling mechanical structures. Even with this much change from the actual form, the hydrodynamic and mechanical behavior of the "cochlea" would be nearly unchanged. The basilar membrane is the yielding structure pictured in Fig. 10. Note that its taper is opposite to that of entire duct. The difference in width is compensated by the spiral lamina. In a long narrow cochlea, fluid flow through the helicotrema would be expected to be negligible except for very low frequencies or to compensate for a static pressure on the stapes. These structures are better identified later in the text

simple understanding of the hydromechanics of the system one ought to remember constantly that the basilar membrane is nearly 100 times as long as its midfrequency width.

Mechanically, the inner ear appears to be best modelled by a hydromechanical transmission line. The input is the plunger-like movement of the footplate of the stapes in the oval window. In response to a sound wave transmitted through the middle ear, the combination of the movement of the stapes and the yielding of the round window creates a time varying pressure difference between the scala vestibuli and the scala tympani, i.e., across the scala media or cochlear duct, whose controlling mechanical element seems to be the basilar membrane.

The hydraulic effect in the cochlea follows a principle called Pascal's law, which says that pressure applied to an enclosed fluid is transmitted undiminished to every portion of the fluid and the walls of the containing vessel. It is this pressure that leads to the yielding of the flexible round window and results in the pressure difference between the scala vestibuli and the scala tympani. The scala media is displaced by this differential pressure. Though it may not be intuitively obvious, the outward pull and the inward push on the stapes lead to a completely symmetrical set of events, i.e., negative pressure effects differ from positive effects only in direction. Thus the displacement of the fluid attributable to the yielding of the round window will follow the time pattern of the applied force at the stapes—or, with the modifications imposed by the transfer function of the middle ear, the force variations impressed by the air on the eardrum.

With this time-varying pressure pattern impressed upon the fluid, the cochlear duct, whose primary supporting structure seems to be the basilar membrane, responds along its length in a very complex manner. Exactly why it does so is still a matter of some argument but it exhibits the traveling wave first observed by von Békésy. The lengthwise pattern to a simple low-frequency sinusoidal pattern can be envisioned by reference to Fig. 9, which shows the instantaneous position of each point on the low-frequency end of the membrane for two moments in time during the passage of the traveling wave. As can be inferred from that portrayal, the amplitude of the wave grows as it travels from base toward helicotrema until it reaches a point most responsive to the particular driving frequency. Past that point, the amplitude of the wave dies rapidly, presumably because of the changing hydromechanical properties of the membrane and the cochlear duct. Fortunately most theorists are convinced that reflections from this point or from the helicotrema are negligible, so we avoid one complicating factor.

In the years following the Békésy observations, a large number of models of the motion of the basilar membrane have appeared. Some have been mechanical, some electrical and some mathematical. But the Békésy measurements are still the only extensive set of observations of the cochlea in action.

In mechanical terminology the basilar membrane behaves as a plate rather than a membrane, since Békésy's additional static measurements show that it is not under tension in either direction. Steele (1974), in fact, models its behavior as a slowly tapering sector of a plate (see Fig. 8) and is able to account for a great deal of its observed motion.

For complex waveforms which contain a small number of frequencies, one can begin to envision the superposition of such patterns along the membrane, but for the spectrally complex and temporally changing waveforms of such useful signals as speech, the pattern of vibration can be very complex indeed.

Reducing the cochlea to two ducts and a boundary between them may be a useful explanatory device for the mechanics of the system, but a glance at Fig. 10 indicates that it may be an unwarranted simplification physiol-

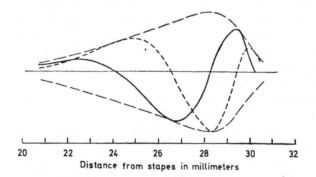

Distance from stapes in millimeters

Fig. 9. Instantaneous position of the membrane at two times during passage of the traveling wave. The membrane is being driven by a 200 Hz tone. At an instant early in one cycle of the wave the membrane is deformed as shown by the dotted line. One quarter cycle later each point will have moved to a new position as shown by the dashed line. What must be kept in mind for a more complete picture is that every point is moving vertically with a sinusoidal motion whose maximum amplitude is indicated by the envelope. As always, it must be borne in mind that the vertical amplitude is greatly exaggerated compared to the horizontal dimension. For an accurate height-length aspect ratio the vertical amplitude would be much less than the thickness of the lines. (From Békésy, 1949)

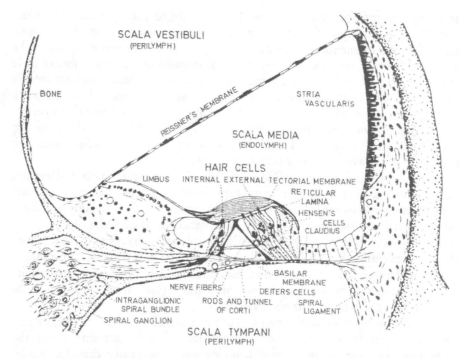

Fig. 10. The structures of the cochlear duct (scala media), showing the complexity of the components that are moved when the basilar membrane is forced into vibration. The surrounding bone is shown as a thin shell because this is the cochlea of a guinea pig. The inner structures are the same as in man. This would be a partial cross section of Fig. 8. The stapes sits at the input end of the scala vestibuli and the round window terminates the scala tympani. Other structures are discussed later in the text. (From Davis *et al.*, 1953)

ogically. As we shall see, we are not yet certain how many of the structures shown have a specific mechanical function, but it is apparent that the cochlear duct is a highly specialized structure. Blood supply to the cochlea, not shown here, is extremely important, since cochlear function deteriorates rapidly when the blood supply is curtailed, and degeneration of structures begins very soon if the blood supply is completely blocked. The arterial supply to the cochlea enters through the internal auditory meatus where the auditory nerve is exiting to the brain stem. One branch of cochlear artery supplies the first quarter to half of the basal turn, the other branch supplies the other turns of the cochlea. From both these branches, one main part of the supply goes to the vascular bed on the outside wall of the cochlea (to the right of Fig. 10) called the *stria vascularis*. This dense bed of capillaries and specialized cells appears to be responsible for secretion of the endolymph, and perhaps also for its reabsorption. *Reissner's membrane*, the very thin membrane that separates the scala media from the scala vestibuli apparently serves no mechanical purpose; it serves rather to separate the two fluids—the perilymph of the scala vestibuli and the endolymph of the scala media—which differ both chemically and electrically. The other boundary of the scala media determines the mechanical behavior of the sensory structures of the cochlea. Parts of that boundary—the *bony spiral lamina*, which lies above and below the exiting nerve fibers, and the *limbus*, the tough fibrous tissue that lies above this spiral lamina—probably are mechanically inert. Steele (1974), however, suggests that at basal locations where the bony shelf is wide, the basilar membrane is comparatively narrow and stiff, and the response is best to high frequencies, vibration of the shelf itself may have some influence. It is also conceivable that the fibrous limbus, in addition to furnishing a relatively fixed mooring for Reissner's membrane and the tectorial membrane, adds enough damping to the bony shelf to which it is attached to keep it from unwanted participation.

Since the basilar membrane is, as suggested previously, the important mechanical structure of the inner ear, structures resting on it do have more directly identifiable functions. Claudius' cells probably furnish some damping for the basilar membrane. Both Deiters' cells and the cells of Hensen appear to be supporting cells for the all-important hair cells. The probable function of the rods of Corti, the reticular lamina and the tectorial membrane will become clearer when we describe the method of stimulation of the nerve fibers at the base of the hair cells.

Fig. 10 also shows quite clearly how the bundle of nerve fibers enters through the spiral lamina. Not shown clearly in that drawing is the fact that each individual fiber enters the fluid of the cochlea through one of the perforations of the bony shelf—*the habenula perforata*. From this point on into the cochlea the fibers no longer have their customary myelin sheath. From that point of entry most of them (95 %) proceed immediately to end on an inner hair cell. Since there are about 3000 inner hair cells to receive nearly 10 times that many nerve fibers, it is not unusual to find many nerve fibers to one inner hair cell. For the outer hair cells, by contrast, since there are less than 2000 fibers to innervate about 9000 cells, one fiber goes to several outer hair cells. These latter fibers wend their way between the arches formed by the rods of Corti, turn basally for a short distance, then branch to terminate on several closely spaced outer hair cells. The reason for this complex innervation pattern is not clear. The cell bodies of these nerve fibers are located in the spiral ganglion, as seen in Fig. 10. The axon portion proceeds on to the cochlear nucleus where we will pick it up in a later discussion.

The two kinds of hair cells are somewhat different in structure and composition, and probably differ in exact function, but we do not as yet have sufficient evidence to spell this out satisfactorily. The outer hair cells are definitely rod or column shaped, whereas the inner hair cells are of a more globular form. Both have sterocilia on the top surface, those on the outer hair cells arranged in the shape of a W with the points toward the outer wall of the cochlea, those on the top of the inner hair cell more nearly in a straight, or slightly curved, line. In both instances, the taller sterocilia make contact with, and may be imbedded in, the tectorial membrane. At the base of the hair cell are the dendritic nerve endings.

The dendritic portion of peripheral nerves—like those found in the fluids of the cochlea ending on the hair cells—is usually stimulated by chemical agents and as a result generates a local, graded electrical current. Under appropriate conditions this triggers the familiar propagated all-or-none response. It is by now sufficiently established that it is the task of the hair cells to furnish the adequate stimulus for the dendritic portion of the peripheral auditory nerves.

How the motion of the structures on the basilar membrane influences the hair cell to stimulate the nerves has been a matter of long conjecture and is still not completely agreed upon. There *is* general agreement that an important pre-neural event is the mechanical distortion of the hair cells. Wever (1971), for example, has traced the methods of hair cell stimulation through many of the vertebrates. In spite of many variations in detail, differential movement between cilia and cell body is consistently the adequate stimulus. Fig. 11 indicates schematically how this might be accomplished (Wever, 1971). According to this scheme, only a few of the inner ear structures are important mechanically. One of these is the tectorial membrane, a comparatively thick gelatinous structure lying above and slightly central to the rows of inner and outer hair cells, and hinged on the spiral limbus. At most audio frequencies this hinge, being over a bony shelf, will not vibrate with the movement of the fluid, so the tectorial membrane has a stationary hinge on its inner edge. In the drawing, the lower edge of the tectorial membrane is the line OC and its extension. Also of mechanical importance are the arches or pillars of Corti which rest on the vibrating part of the basilar membrane. These are represented by the legs of triangle o′ab. At the top of the pillars is the reticular membrane composed of a tough connective tissue, forming a mosaic around the tops of the hair cells, with the hairs projecting upward toward, and possibly into, the bottom of the tectorial membrane. When point b of the basilar membrane moves downward further than point o′, the reticular

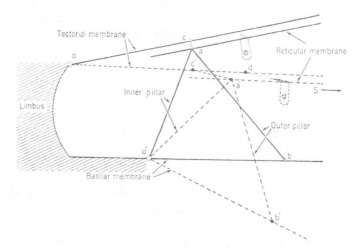

Fig. 11. Diagram of a possible method for bending the hairs at the top of the hair cells. It is admittedly greatly exaggerated for purposes of illustration. See the text for explanation and Fig. 10 for the shape of the structures involved. (From Wever, 1971)

plate—and with it the top of the hair cell—is pushed much further from the upper point of attachment of the hair(s) than it was in the position of rest (o'ab). Where the hair was originally upright, it is now sharply bent.

This is a persuasive pattern for the occurrence of shear-like motions of the structure associated with the hair cells. One needs to remember, in assessing the validity of such an explanation, that it must be plausible at threshold amplitudes as well as the extreme example shown here. Modern measurements suggest that the lowest effective amplitudes of movement of the basilar membrane are of the order of a fraction of an Ångstrom. By way of orientation to this somewhat different order of movement, the length of a hair cell is 60,000 Ångstroms (6 microns). Although the explanation is an attractive one, operation at sub-Ångstrom amplitudes still calls for keeping an open mind.

Whatever the correct explanation, movement of the basilar membrane and associated structures is coincident with impulses in the fibers of the VIIIth nerve. The highly complex cochlea is much more than a mechanical amplifier. From the orientation of the nerves to the hair cells, we are looking in the right place, but the explanation is far from complete. Which aspect of the complicated motion we have looked at thus far actually triggers a nerve impulse?

Electric Potential in the Cochlea

The electrical behavior of the cochlea has been a topic of interest, measurement and discussion by auditory physiologists for nearly 50 years. The question of whether the cochlear transformation from mechanical events to neural pattern is best understood through electrical or chemical phenomena is currently a highly pertinent one. Whichever is eventually the most fruitful orientation, the measurement of electrical potentials and electrical changes in the cochlea has been one of the most revealing endeavors in our study of cochlear operation.

Perhaps the most useful of these electric cochlear potentials is the one known as the cochlear microphonic (CM). As the name implies, one of the potentials measurable in the cochlea suggests that the cochlea behaves as a microphone in the sense that it creates an electrical wave that has the same waveform as the mechanical motion of the cochlea. Since it is an electric potential it can be picked up anywhere inside the cochlea, but exploration with suitable electrodes has shown it to be strongest in the immediate vicinity of the hair cells.

Closer study of the electric behavior of the cochlea shows that there is also a constant (DC) voltage difference of +80 mv between the fluid in the scala media and that in scala tympani. Inside the hair cell, on the other hand, the potential measures —60 mv referred to the same point in the perilymph. Davis (1978) has a very reasonable electrical analog for the function of these

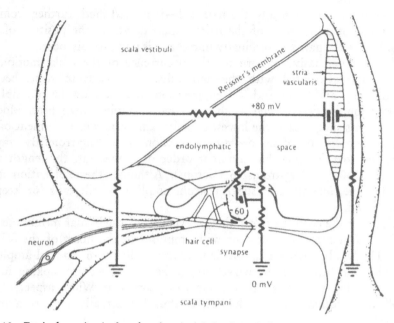

Fig. 12. Equivalent circuit for the electrical behavior of the cochlea superimposed on the cochlear structure. The single hair cell shown represents both the inner and outer hair cells. The shunt paths shown are recognition of the fact that there will inevitably be leakage from the positive or negative voltage points through other tissue paths to the neutral (reference) point. For the understanding of the electrical operation of the cochlea these paths can be ignored. See the text for further explanation. (From Davis, 1978)

voltages, related to the cochlea as shown in Fig. 12. Following his analogy, the stria vascularis performs as a battery to keep the potential of the endolymph at 80 mv above the neutral, unpolarized portions of the body fluids. The hair cell represents electrically an oppositely polarized battery, and the sum of these two (140 mv) appears across the top, hair-bearing portion of the hair cell. According to Davis, some part or element at the top of the hair cell may behave electrically like the variable resistance shown between the two batteries. Mechanical deformation of the cell leads to a change in resistance, thence to a change in current through the hair cell, and this in turn mediates the level of polarization at the base of the cell. The release of a chemical mediator to excite the afferent nerve ending at the base of the cell is controlled by this level of polarization. This makes the cochlear microphonic, essentially an alternating current resulting from modulation of the DC potential, a vital link in the chain from mechanical to neural processing by the cochlea. Whether the causal connection is as close as this model suggests or whether the cochlear microphonic is more nearly epiphenomenal to more directly chemically mediated events is not important to our present understanding of cochlear operation. Whichever is the case, electrical measurement of preneural cochlear events continues to be an important means of assessing behavior, subject to the precautions that should always be observed when our understanding is incomplete.

Cochlear Innervation

We may infer from Fig. 10 that two columns of hair cells are arrayed down the length of the cochlea, one on either side of the arches of Corti. The inner hair cells form in single file, as it were, and the outer in rows of three. We have noted that inner and outer hair cells are different in form and that the pattern of hairs at the top is distinctly different in the two types. This contrast in hair pattern and in mechanical placement has been well noted by both physiologists and mechanical modelers of the cochlea.

It is possible in experimental animals to destroy the outer hair cells, leaving the inner intact. Analysis of the resulting changes in microphonic and in neural firing pattern has led to some provocative conjecture about difference in function, particularly by Zwislocki and his co-workers (Zwislocki and Sokolich, 1974; Zwislocki and Kletsky, 1979). But we do not really know the detailed motion of the structures well enough to say confidently how they might differ basically in their mechanical function. They definitely do differ in their pattern of innervation, and the pattern is not what one would predict from the way the cells are arrayed.

The total count of hair cells in the two rows is about 12,000. The inner hair cells, slightly larger than the outer ($\sim$ 10 microns), number about 3000; the remaining 9000 are in the three rows of outer hair cells. The single row of inner hair cells runs about 100 cells per mm, and the outer rows roughly 100 rows of three. They are, in other words, closely packed in the longitudinal dimension. Since we have already seen that this is the dimension where frequency differences are separated, this hair-cell spacing should be of special interest. In the frequency range where frequency discrimination is best the smallest frequency difference that makes a difference in perceived pitch corresponds to a spacing along the basilar membrane smaller than the 10 μ spacing between hair cells.

Paralleling the rows of hair cells along the spiral of the cochlea is a row of nerve cell bodies just central to the scala media. This is the spiral ganglion and these are cell bodies of bi-polar nerve units which send dendrites to the hair cells in the cochlea and axons to the cochlear nucleus.

The pattern of innervation of the hair cells is neatly shown in a diagram from Spoendlin (1975) reproduced here in Fig. 13. This is actually from the cochlea of the cat, but there is little reason to suppose the pattern is different for the human cochlea. The left block of the diagram shows the course of the afferent neurons, with their cell bodies between the dotted lines labeled sg (spiral ganglion). Each inner hair cell receives a number of dendrites directly from the cell bodies of the spiral ganglion. This, as shown, accounts for 95 % of all afferent neurons, which could be as many as 27,000 units. The remaining 5 % go mostly to the outer hair cells as shown. The break in the middle of the diagram indicates that each of these latter fibers, on its way to synapsing with about 10 outer hair cells in the manner shown, passes under the outer hair cells (through the Deiters cells of Fig. 10) for about 0.6 mm—about 100 cells.

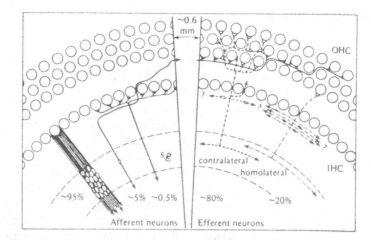

Fig. 13. The pattern of neural connections in the cochlea. Each block on either side of the 0.6 mm gap showns a span of about 0.1 mm with one connection of each kind shown. Further detail in the text. (From Spoendlin, 1975)

The right-hand block of Fig. 13 shows the pattern of innervation of the efferent fibers to the cochlea. There are a total of about 500 of these fibers. Virtually nothing of their function has been established with any certainty. In contrast to the afferent fibers they go almost exclusively to outer hair cells. They have been traced from cortex down to the superior olivary nucleus (see Fig. 19), the locus of the cell bodies for these efferent fibers to the cochlea. They are the object of considerable curiosity and conjecture, but for our purposes it seems wisest to note their presence and pass on.

Frequency Analysis in the Cochlea   4

It would seem axiomatic that if the sense of hearing is to be useful rapid vibrations (high frequency sounds) should give a different sensation than slow vibrations (low frequency sounds). We saw in our early view of the pattern of the traveling wave in Fig. 9 that this frequency separation begins in the cochlea. A more detailed view can be constructed from measuring the electrical response (cochlear microphonic) at a number of points. This looks like the curves in Fig. 14 (Eldredge, 1978).

The fact that the dispersion of the pattern of excitation along the membrane can be read from the output of the VIIIth nerve is shown by some painstaking work of Pfeiffer and Kim (1975) on individual fibers in the VIIIth nerve of the cat. The results are portrayed in Fig. 15. To understand these graphs we may begin with the bottom display marked 3600 Hz. This indicates that for all the data taken for this lowest panel, the cochlea was

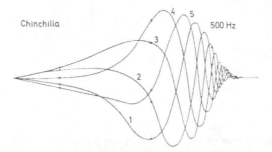

Fig. 14. An estimate of the amplitude pattern of the traveling wave derived from the amplitude of the cochlear microphonic in the cochlea of the chinchilla. Several animals have a thin wall around a cochlea that protrudes from the temporal bone, making easier access to desired locations on the membrane. These measurements have been taken at three widely spaced points, with the cochlea driven at 500 Hz. The 5 curves are equally spaced in time through the 2 msec period of the driving wave. Recent observations of the response of single points on the membrane suggest the envelope may have a sharper peak than is implied here.
(From Eldredge, 1974)

being driven with a 3600 Hz sinusoid. Each plotted dot represents performance of a separate fiber under this driving condition. Its horizontal placement
is determined by the best, or characteristic, frequency of that fiber—the one

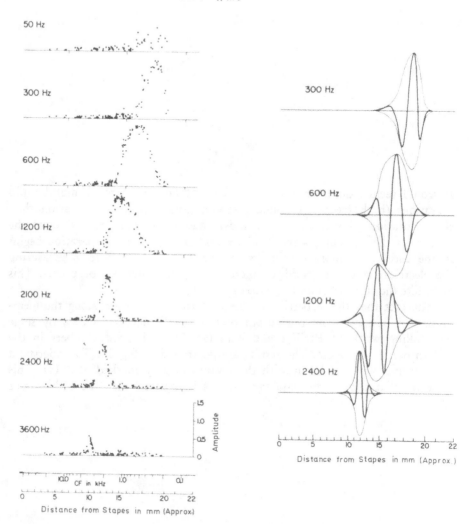

Fig. 15. Left: The pattern of response of different VIIIth nerve fibers to a pure tone. Each
plotted point represents a fiber. Horizontal position of the point is determined by its characteristic frequency. Vertical placement depends on its rate of firing in response to the tone. The
tones were presented at 20 dB SPL, except for the 50 Hz tone, which had to be increased to
60 dB SPL for sufficient response. Right: The plots of A have been used to derive amplitude
envelopes at certain frequencies of the implied basilar membrane vibration pattern. Inside
this envelope is the shape of the traveling wave (heavy line) for one instant of time, that
instant being the moment when the peak of the wave was at the peak of the envelope. If rate
of nerve response can be taken to be proportional to basilar membrane amplitude, these are
good estimates of the traveling wave envelope at low level. (From Pfeiffer and Kim, 1975)

to which it shows the lowest threshold. The relation of the distance and characteristic frequency (CF) scale along the abscissa is derived from many previous experiments on the frequency effects of injury at different points in the cat cochlea. The vertical placement of the dot is derived from the total number of discharges from that unit in a standard time.

It is apparent that as a unit's characteristic frequency departs further from the driving frequency its rate of response is lower. On the reasonable assumption that rate of responding is related to membrane amplitude, we are seeing an indication of the amplitude pattern of the membrane. Pfeiffer and Kim proceeded to derive traveling wave shapes from these implied amplitude patterns. These, as shown in Fig. 15, are very useful if we remember again that the vertical-horizontal aspect ratio is completely arbitrary. To attempt a realistic image of the amplitude pattern one must remember that the amplitude for these patterns, for which the driving wave was 20 dB Sound Pressure Level, would be at best a few Ångstroms and therefore not visible under our best microscopes. The hair cells which read this pattern are truly amazing devices.

Even at these low levels, that pattern, however, is rather broad; and even our unaided auditory intuition tells us that better frequency separation must take place further on in the system. Just what or where the difference in pattern may be for eventually perceiving that one sound has a different frequency than another is not known, but already at the output of the cochlea it is apparent some narrowing of the pattern has occurred. For some years now neurophysiologists have been able to record the responses (action potentials) from individual neurons for different frequencies in such animals as cats, guinea pigs or monkeys. One kind of frequency response, or "tuning curve" for a typical first-order auditory neuron looks like the solid line of Fig. 16. In order to understand this graph, the method of measurement is important. Having succeeded in placing a microelectrode (1 micron or less in diameter)

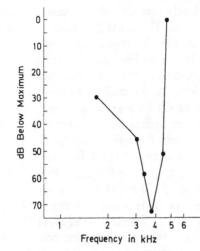

Fig. 16. The response area of a VIIIth nerve fiber.
See the text for its derivation

on a single nerve fiber, the experimenter acquaints himself with both the auditory and visible "feel" of the fibre. What this means is that each first-order neuron fires spontaneously in the absence of an external signal, and what the experimenter is looking for as evidence of the earliest (lowest level) response of that fiber is a change in the pattern of firing when the external signal is applied. So the experimenter listens to the pattern of spontaneous firing and looks at it on an oscilloscope trace, then applies a very weak external signal, varying its frequency over the range of interest until at some frequency a change in pattern can be discerned. Next, the level of the signal is raised, and the same process repeated. What is recorded on the graph of Fig. 16 for each level of the signal is the range of frequencies for which the neuron departed from its spontaneous firing pattern. Note that each fiber shows this change at only a single frequency (its best, or characteristic frequency) when the applied signal is at its weakest. As the signal is made stronger, the range of response grows wider, but not very rapidly so that it appears that the response of the fiber has a sharper frequency response than does the point on the basilar membrane with which the fiber is associated. This presents a puzzle we will look at shortly. Meantime, note that other fibers shown on the graph with different characteristic frequencies have similar response shapes. We might note also for later reference that the range of frequencies over which the fiber responds does not spread symmetrically as the signal is increased, but spreads more toward the low frequencies. This is suggested, but certainly not predicted precisely from the form of the traveling wave shown in Fig. 14. If we drove the stapes with a lower frequency the excitation pattern would move to the right, and the point which previously had been responding with greatest amplitude would still be moving with considerable amplitude. But if we shifted to a higher frequency and the pattern moved to the left the amplitude at our chosen point would drop, though perhaps not so precipitously as the high-frequency end of the tuning curve.

Though such graphs as Fig. 16 have long been referred to as tuning curves, the technique does not closely resemble the process of measuring the frequency response of any other device. The usual procedure would be to keep the input to the device constant across the frequency range of interest and note the changes in the output. If we follow this procedure with our neuron being recorded by the microelectrode, we may get plots that look like those in Fig. 17. Here the input level to the cochlea has been held constant at the SPL indicated by the number of dB on a given contour and the measure of output is taken as number of nerve spikes per unit time from the fiber in question. Note that the spontaneous rate from this fiber (at the lower right) is very low. As the stimulation level is changed from low to high the response pattern roughly resembles what we might predict from Fig. 14. For frequencies lower than its "best frequency" of 2100 Hz the unit responds more frequently than it does for higher frequencies. This is not true for the fiber response plotted in B. Looking at a larger sample of fibers, Rose *et al.* (1971) saw many variations of these two plots, but in general the top plot portrays the type of response from fibers with high best frequency and the bottom from those with low best frequency.

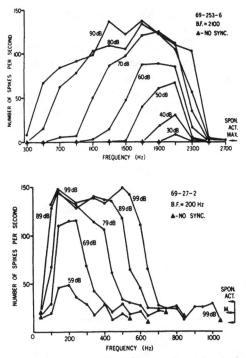

Fig. 17. The change in response rate of a fiber as intensity is held constant and the frequency varies as shown on the abscissa. The arrows at the right indicate the range of spontaneous rates and the mean spontaneous rate of discharge. B.F. indicates best frequency of the fiber. In many measurements, the top pattern is typical of fibers with high characteristic frequency, and the bottom of fibers with low CF. (From Rose *et al.*, 1971)

But the situation is complicated somewhat further by the fact that fibers of the VIIIth nerve exhibit a *range* of spontaneous discharge rates. In Fig. 18 is shown the plot of the output-rate response of a fiber with a very high spontaneous rate. Its response appears to differ very little across the range of input frequencies. However, if we record only those output spikes that are synchronized with the input, *i.e.*, that are spaced by the period of the driving frequency as in the lower graph, we get an entirely different notion of how response differs at different frequencies.

When this fiber is responding to a very soft tone (35 dB SPL) at its best frequency almost all of the response spikes are synchronized to the driving frequency, but at adjacent frequencies very few of them are. Such a fiber could be very useful for detecting a change in firing pattern in the presence of weak signals or for aiding other (adjacent) fibers in the fine discrimination of frequency differences.

Even this sketchy look at the behavior of first order neurons poses an interesting question. In further processing, does the system look at the dispersion pattern of units that are responding, as suggested by the shape of the envelope of Fig. 15; does it read some pattern of strength of output, as from the data of Fig. 17; or does it make more specific use of the synchrony of different simultaneously responding units? Considering the overall versatility of the system, the answer probably will be that it makes use of all of such aspects of the responding pattern.

In our discussion of Fig. 16 we noted that first-order neurons appear to have a sharper tuning curve than the point on the membrane where the nerve is situated. This has led a number of theorists to conjecture that there may be some additional tuning between the mechanical behavior of the membrane and the firing of the nerve. Russell and Sellick (1978) succeeded in

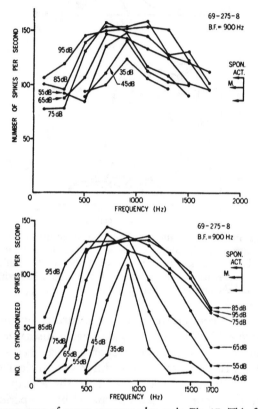

Fig. 18. Top: The same type of nerve-response plot as in Fig. 17. This fiber has a very high spontaneous rate. Bottom: For this plot of the response of the same fiber the only spikes counted are those that are synchronized with the driving frequency. How sensitive the following auditory system is to synchronous discharges rather than simply total discharges per unit time is a matter of great interest. (From Rose et al., 1971)

getting a microelectrode inside one of the inner hair cells of a guinea pig. From a number of such cell preparations, they recorded the DC voltage response for signals of different frequency and showed that by this measure the cell exhibits as sharp tuning as the response recorded for nerve fibers. This makes it appear that some aspect of the motion of the membrane does exhibit sharper tuning than the amplitude envelope as usually observed. Many students of the auditory process, following von Békésy's lead (1953) believe it is some facet of the shear motion on the hair cells as described by Ter Kuile and Wever. (See Fig. 17.)

Central Auditory System 5

How is it that these spike-like signals from thousands of cochlear nerve fibers eventually enable the organism to perceive the myriad sounds of the environment? Auditory signals must present nearly as complex a problem for processing as visual patterns, since they are highly transitory in nature and cover a huge dynamic range. Perhaps for this reason, the auditory brainstem itself seems a complicated network. A highly simplified scheme showing at least the basic serial path traversed by impulses that originate at the cochlea appears in Fig. 19. It is indeed the simplest of portrayals, since at each level not only are there many parallel connections within that level, but in addition connections to other, non-auditory areas become important.

Greater structural detail than this would presumably be of only limited interest to anyone except auditory physiologists and neurologists.

We can probably anticipate increasing complexity of analysis with increasing distance from the cochlea since the number of units presumably assigned to auditory processing increases rapidly as we progress further up the auditory tract. In the monkey Chow (1951) has estimated that there are 190,000 cells in the cochlear nucleus, 400,000 at the level of the medial geniculate and 10,000,000 at the cortex. Add to this the fact that at each level there are outputs to motor systems and connections to other sensory systems.

We know at this point (1980) very little about the locus of specific functions along this pathway or indeed whether we should look for specific loci for known auditory processes. Nevertheless, it seems useful to note the major anatomical features before attempting to discuss the kind of functions that might reasonably be established.

All of the fibers traveling centrally from the spiral ganglion of the cochlea terminate somewhere in the complex of the cochlear nucleus. Whereas the fibers of the VIIIth nerve all behave essentially similarly, there is great variety in the response of different fibers within the cochlear nucleus. The fibers branch in such a way that the geometric layout of the cochlea is represented in at least three separate places. Wherever these ordered frequency

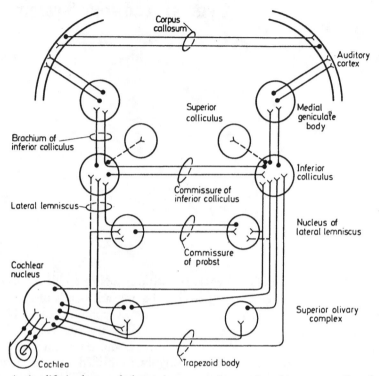

Fig. 19. A simplified scheme of the major connections and pathways ascending from the cochlea to the cortex. Connections are shown from only one cochlea. Dashed lines indicate paths not completely verified. (From Neff, 1975)

representations occur throughout the auditory brainstem and the cortex, they are referred to as tonotopic. This may well mean, however, that tonal frequency is the dimension most easily identified that corresponds to the geometric configuration of the cochlea. To a degree, point to point representation of peripheral areas in central neural complexes is the rule throughout the central nervous system. It seems more useful, then, to designate such cochlear alignments as *cochleotopic* until we know more of the specific purpose for any one of them.

At the cochlear nucleus is the first level where conventional neural inhibition is possible. A pattern that is operationally indistinguishable from inhibition appears also in primary auditory neurons, and we discuss it in the section on cochlear frequency analysis. This process of creating contrast by a subtraction-like analysis is only one of the modifications taking place even at this early level. Using fairly specifiable signals, like tone bursts, clicks and click trains, two-tone combinations, amplitude- and frequency-modulated tone, ascending and descending frequency ramps and amplitude modulated noise, it has been possible to classify the response of cochlear nucleus units into at least 9 different types. Thus it seems apparent that this nucleus is much more than a straightforward relay station. Individual units of the cochlear nucleus show as wide a range of spontaneous discharge rates as do those of the cochlear nerve, but there the close similarity seems to end. Only about 10 % of these units exhibit response patterns resembling those of the primary units in the VIIIth nerve.

As can be seen in Fig. 19 axons from the cochlear nucleus travel contralaterally to end in the lateral lemniscus and the inferior colliculus. Others go to the superior olivary complex, some to the same side, some contralaterally, through the trapezoid body. At the olivary complex is the earliest meeting of innervation from both cochleas, and it appears this complex is involved in processing the fine interaural time differences that permit localization of sound sources (Masterton and Diamond, 1967). At least until recently, it was probably the most thoroughly worked area of the auditory brainstem. Typically what takes place here is that spikes arriving from one cochlea will inhibit those arriving from the other. It happens particularly when the signals from one ear lead those from the other in time, but we shall see in our discussion of binaural hearing that the time-frequency-intensity pattern between ears can differ in intricate ways and the analysis must be highly complicated. Sound oriented reflexes, such as the contraction of middle ear muscles and the eye blink in response to sudden onset of loud sounds, also appear to be controlled at this early level, probably because speed of response is highly important.

Up to the level of the trapezoid body, when the input to the cochlea is a click the response of many units is more than one spike and these are spaced, as they are at the cochlea, by a period that is the reciprocal of the characteristic frequency of the unit. This can hold for best frequencies as high as 3 kc (Goldberg, 1975). It represents unusual preservation of time relations across synapses. Furthermore, Evans (1975) remarks that phaselocking, the tendency for a unit to fire at the same phase point in later cycles of the driving frequency (even though it will seldom fire on adjacent cycles), persists over large level changes, i.e., it may occur over changes from 10 to 90 dB above "threshold". And Goldstein and Abeles (1975) point out that even though this phase locking may be shown by fewer cells as we move centrally, it has been reported up to the inferior colliculus. The importance of timing is evident throughout the auditory system.

In contrast to the superior olive, very little of the innervation of the lateral lemniscus is binaural. Most neurons here are affected only by stimulation of the contralateral ear. As with the cochlear nucleus, there is a wide variety of response among the units, and in some units the pattern of response may differ greatly according to the intensity or frequency of the stimulating tone. These units are undoubtedly influenced by inputs from several lower levels.

The inferior colliculus receives innervation from both sides; but as is apparent in Fig. 19, this innervation may arrive by a number of paths and from a number of levels—some as peripheral as the contralateral cochlear nucleus. As we move further up the system it might be reasonable to expect that input signals of greater complexity will be required to deduce how or whether the system responds differently to different kinds of signals. At the inferior colliculus, for instance, very few cells responded when the input to the cochlea was a steady-state pure tone, but by the use of modulated signals, Erulkar, Nelson and Bryant (1968) revealed that some cells respond to a frequency sweep in only one direction, others to only the opposite, and that some cells which respond to amplitude modulation respond only when the modulation reaches a certain rate. These are relatively simple signals compared with speech, music or many of the meaningful sounds of the environment, and only from many, many such analyses could we hope to deduce in what specific way(s) the function of the inferior colliculus might differ from areas either higher or lower in the ascending auditory system. As is apparent in the diagram, the colliculus receives a varied input, so that integration of partial processing from other levels might well be expected at this locus.

The medial geniculate body can be seen to be the last area in the ascending path to the cortex. It also receives input *from* the cortex on many of the dendrites of its principal cells. Interestingly enough, there are no crossings at this level—only interaction with higher and lower levels; and in some parts inputs from the somato-sensory system. The medial geniculate sends a point to point projection to area AI, a primary auditory area, in the cortex.

As might be predicted, if processing at this level represents an advanced stage, only rarely does one encounter continued response to sustained tones. The more usual response to such static signals is an onset burst followed by silence. Harris (1974) conjectures that, because some units show cyclic spontaneous activity and some unusually large latencies, this area is adapted for storage of time patterns that are to be analyzed in something slower than real time.

For purely practical reasons, the method of studying the auditory network is to find a single unit whose activity can be recorded and present a variety of inputs to the cochlea, noting the response of the unit for each type of input. Ideally, one might prefer a closer imitation of what we must suppose is the method of physiological interpretation, that is, presenting a signal of interest and viewing simultaneously a sufficiently large sample of neural units to see changes in pattern paralleling a change in the stimulus. The shortcomings of the practical method are much more apparent at the upper levels of auditory processing—perhaps particularly at the cortex.

The auditory physiologist encounters an additional problem at this level because most experiments must be done on anesthetized animals. This means that measures made in the higher levels of the system are highly suspect, and this, too, has slowed the accumulation of such information as can be gleaned about the function of the cortex.

In addition, even though we may consider clicks, modulated tones, spectrally and temporally shaped noises, etc., to be more suitable stimuli than easily specified tones, they are still far removed from the signals in the environment that might reasonably by expected to engage the analyzing capabilities of the central stages of analysis. Thus work on the cortex, although of extreme interest and importance, has proceeded slowly and the emerging picture is fragmentary.

Some of the types of response characteristic of lower levels are still present—usually less prevalent—at the cortex. Restricted frequency response can still be shown for some units, for example, the inhibition of one tone by another simultaneous one and the inhibitory interaction of inputs from the two sides. Although phase locking to tones has not been found at the cortical level, time locking to click trains has been reported, even to trains as fast as 1000/sec, though presumably few cells will follow this rate (Rouiller *et al.*, 1979).

We have spoken of the auditory cortex as though it were a single area. Such is not the case. The auditory cortex of the cat comprises the areas shown in Fig. 20. Most of the findings suggested here came from work on area AI, since very little single-unit recording has been done from other areas. Presumably the total cortical area actually associated with audition in man is even more complex considering his activities in such areas as speech and music not shared to any significant degree by the cat.

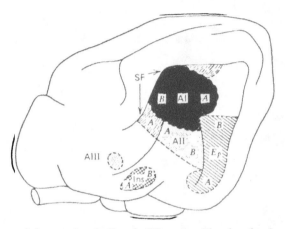

Fig. 20. The cortex of the cat. Areas *AI* and *AII* are considered to be the primary auditory areas in the cat cortex. Projections from these areas go to the other areas identified. *Ep* posterior ectosylvian; *Ins* Insular region; *SF* suprasylvian fringe. *A* and *B* refer to apex and base of the cochlea, the origin for the areas marked. (From Woolsey, 1960)

Part II
Psychoacoustics

We turn now from an introduction to the anatomy and physiology of the auditory mechanism to a consideration of the system's response to a variety of standard signals. It is convenient to consider sounds as varying basically in frequency, intensity, duration and spectral and temporal complexity. How the auditory perceptual response differs as changes are made in these fundamental aspects of sounds encompasses much of the study of psychoacoustics. It would be comforting, of course, if we could tie each of the findings back to some facet of the physiology or neurophysiology of the system. This is possible only in a few instances, and then quite indirectly.

The psychoacoustic method of investigating the auditory system is fundamentally different from the physiological. The physiologist can be frustrated by the fact that the species available to him have few of the interesting auditory capabilities of the human. In a sense there are *too many* discrete outputs available and only a pictorial diagram available to work from rather than even a good functional block diagram. The only technique available to the psychoacoustician, on the other hand, is to anticipate what set of signals and signal changes at the input to the system will serve to assess the system's behavior and to measure systematically the responses at the output. Two of the major problems with this approach are the fact that there are too many stages between the input and the only output available to us—we have no intermediate test points—and the additional fact that the auditory output, meaning our repertoire of descriptive terms for the sounds we hear, is a highly restricted one. Worse still, many of these descriptive terms are used consensually by only small groups.

One reason for this latter situation is that we seldom, in our everyday interchange, have occasion to discuss sounds as they are used in the psychoacoustic laboratory. The function of the auditory system is to convert sound into forms useful to the listening organism. Our responses consist primarily of recognition of sound sources and what they are doing, and only indirectly of judgements of pitch, loudness, duration, etc., of sounds. As a consequence, most of what we have learned in the psychoacoustic laboratory has been pieced together by doing experiments that limit the listener's answer to such judgements as louder-softer, higher-lower, same-different; or measuring such indirect responses as reaction time to differing input signals. This is good science in the sense of imposing quantifiability, and sometimes repeatability. But it also imposes the additional burden of a considerable amount of extrapolation beyond the findings themselves in building a model for comprehensive understanding of the auditory system.

The implication of this state of affairs for the study of the auditory system by current psychoacoustic methods, is that we are studying only a restricted part of the system, and that frequently the output available to us is rather far removed from the point in the system where basic correlates of such fundamental dimensions as those mentioned above are determined.

These reservations are voiced here not to foster a lack of faith in the psychoacoustic study of the auditory system, but rather to explicate—perhaps to justify—the incomplete state of our analysis of the total system; and even more importantly to advocate appropriate patience in the interpretation, and particularly in the extrapolation, of findings that, at our present stage of understanding, must be subject to modification until we have filled in more of the vacant slots in a complete model of auditory processing.

Auditory Sensitivity 6

Sensory systems are admirably efficient in the sense that they detect astonishingly small quantities of the information they are tailored to respond to. In vision, audition and smell, these systems rival in sensitivity the achievements of modern technology. When we speak of measuring the minimum sensitivity of the auditory system we talk about amounts of energy and amplitudes of motion which are almost impossible to grasp intuitively. Within the last decade it has been possible to measure the behavior of the mechanical part of the system at something approaching its normal operating amplitudes of around 10 Å, using laser interferometer techniques (Tonndorf and Khanna, 1972). Transfer of these amplitudes to those of the basilar membrane and extrapolation from these measurements down to minimum operating levels (threshold) has essentially confirmed the original extrapolation of von Békésy that minimum basilar membrane amplitudes in the sensitive mid-frequency range of the ear are about 10^{-2} Å. Fortunately, the signal at the eardrum which creates this basilar membrane amplitude is still 18 dB above the Brownian noise amplitude of the air at the drum; and the inherent Brownian noise of the cochlea has an energy about 22 dB down from the minimum energy required for threshold at the hair cell (Harris, 1968).

One should not get the impression that this degree of sensitivity obtains over the entire frequency range. It is only in the ear's most sensitive range that such extremely small amplitudes are sufficient to influence the spontaneous firing pattern of the VIIIth nerve enough to create a perception of sound. How the level of signal needed for a pure tone to be audible about half the time varies over the audible frequency range is shown in Fig. 21. If we look at the various curves it is apparent that what we take as minimally audible depends to some extent on how it was measured, since the curves for different conditions and methods differ in placement. In general, however, all curves indicate increasing sensitivity as we progress from very low frequencies toward the middle of the range. The maximum sensitivity lies in the range from about 800 Hz to possibly 4 kHz. This is also the primary range in which speech

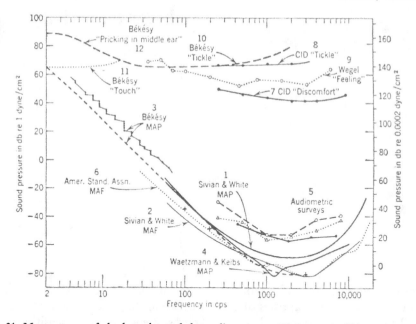

Fig. 21. Measurement of the boundary of the auditory area. Minimum Audible Field (*MAF*) measurements are made without earphone; Minimum Audible Pressure (*MAP*) indicates measures with phones. Curves marked 5 were not taken in as quiet environments as other minimum sensitivity curves. Curve 6 is a compilation of MAP measurements. Both upper and lower borders vary depending on how and where the measurements are made. See the text for a description of the decibel scale. (From Licklider, 1951)

sounds differ most from each other. How nearly this may not be fortuitous is difficult to assess, but the fact remains that Man produces sound best in the range where his auditory system receives it most efficiently.

The ordinate on the graph is essentially the logarithm of the pressure variation in the air which gives rise to a sound strong enough to be audible by the criterion given earlier. This particular logarithmic scale is in decibels (dB) a unit converting the pressure or energy ratio of two sounds into the difference between their logarithms,

$$\text{Difference in dB} = 10 \log \frac{E_1}{E_2} = 20 \log \frac{P_1}{P_2}$$

and thus scaling down the tremendous energy range over which the ear operates to more manageable numbers. When the specific scale is the one used here, Sound Pressure Level[1], the denominator of the ratio on the right of the

---

[1] The Sound Pressure Level of a sound in dB is defined as

$$\text{SPL}_{dB} = 20 \log \frac{P_s}{P_{ref}}$$

where P_{ref} is the reference for the SPL scale.

P_{ref} in the older literature is given as 2×10^{-4} dynes/cm² which is 2 dynes/m² and therefore the same as 20 microPascals since 1 Pascal is 1 Newton/m² and 1 dyne = 10^{-5} Newton.

equation is the reference pressure variation—an rms amplitude of 20 μPa. This was originally thought to be the minimum pressure variation detectable by the auditory system in its most sensitive range, but the measurements shown in the figure indicate that under ideal listening conditions the minimum may be even lower. This makes no problem in the setting of reference levels, since a sound with 1/10 the energy of the reference sound still differs by 10 dB and therefore has a Sound Pressure Level of —10 dB.

We have remarked about the impressive sensitivity of the ear, but it is also remarkable for the intensity *range* over which it operates. The ratio between the pressure required to make a tone just barely audible in the middle range and the pressure at which the tone becomes unbearably strong is over a million to one—a decibel difference of more than 120. This usable range gets smaller as the frequency goes lower, but even at around 100 Hz, the low frequency range for musical instruments and the fundamental frequency for low-pitched male voices, the range is still better than 60 dB.

Minimum Audible Pressure

Traditionally, there are two methods for leading sound to the ear for measuring minimum audible sound. The most common one in the laboratory and in the audiology clinic is to have an earphone on the ear. At some frequency, say 1000 Hz, the level from the earphone is varied according to some predetermined routine until one discovers the level detected by the listener on half of the listening trials. The sound pressure level (dB difference from 20 μPa) at the eardrum is called the Minimum Audible Pressure (MAP) for that frequency. How does one measure the sound pressure at the eardrum? The most accurate method available is to insert a small probe tube, whose effect on the sound reaching the drum is negligible and whose effect on the sound it transmits is also known at each frequency of interest, and lead that probe tube to a calibrated microphone.

A less valid measure, but acceptable for many purposes and much more convenient, is to record the voltage driving the earphone and then to place the earphone on a standard coupler. This coupler has closely specified dimensions and terminates in a calibrated laboratory microphone. The calibration data on the microphone yields the value of the sound pressure level in the coupler. Because the ear is so sensitive, these procedures are seldom used for measurement of minimum levels, but are used whenever there is occasion to estimate sound pressure at the eardrum delivered by an earphone and extrapolated to threshold when desired.

Minimum Audible Field

The second laboratory method for delivering sound under controlled conditions is via loudspeaker. In this case, the method of specifying sound delivered to the ears is to place the calibrated microphone at the position of the center of the listener's head. The level barely audible to the listener has already been established. The listener is removed from the field, the loudspeaker is driven at some known level above that just audible (by some formal criterion), and again the output of the calibrated microphone, at the position occupied by the listener's head, gives by extrapolation the value of the minimum audible sound.

In the middle range, if these measurements are made carefully with the probe tube method rather than with the coupler (MAP) or the microphone substitution (MAF) method, the sound pressure at the eardrum when the listener can detect the presence of the tone correctly half the time is the same whether the signal is being delivered by the earphone or the loudspeaker. At low frequencies, however, the sound pressure level (SPL) may be as much as 6 dB lower for the loudspeaker case than for sound from the earphone. There is some evidence (see Shaw, 1974, p. 486) that the difference comes about because the earphone on the ear creates a cavity that enhances the physiological noises of the body (breathing, blood flow, blood pumping, even muscular activity). Remember that we are considering very low level signals in speaking of absolute sensitivity. Attempts to measure the noise occasioned by even minimal normal physiological activity indicate its level and the shape of its spectrum is about right for interfering with minimum audible signals, as shown in Fig. 22. This would be very interesting since we would then suppose that the explanation for at least part of the shape of the sensitivity curve of the ear, as shown in Fig. 20, lies in the spectrum of this physiological noise. However, the fact that the signal delivered by a loudspeaker above threshold is louder than a signal from an earphone when the two are creating the same sound pressure at the eardrum makes it difficult to accept the interference, or

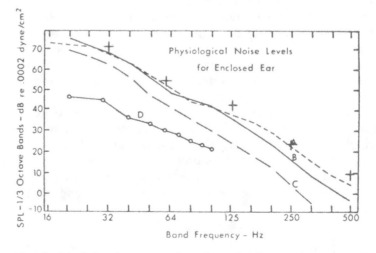

Fig. 22. The physiological noise measured at the enclosed ears of human subjects. The different curves come from different kinds of enclosing cavities, but the +'s marking the average threshold at certain frequencies show that such levels may interfere with sensitivity measurement. This will become clearer in Chapter 10, when it is shown that the noise in about a ¹/₃-octave band surrounding a tone contributes most of the interference (masking) for that tone. (From Shaw, 1974)

masking, explanation of the discrepancy between earphone and loudspeaker reception.

Anderson and Whittle (1971) presented listeners a tone of the same frequency (125 Hz) alternately coming from a phone and a loudspeaker. The listeners were instructed to balance the tones in loudness. When the two tones were judged equally loud, the sound pressure level at the drum was lower for the tone from the speaker than for the phone. This difference diminished as the tones were made stronger, but did not disappear until the SPL reached 80 dB. This is about 40 dB above the measured threshold at that frequency.

Another possibility for explaining the difference is that at these frequencies the exchange of energy between air and ear is better when the open ear canal receives energy from the air than when it is part of an enclosure. This is to say that there is a better impedance match between eardrum and open canal than between drum and occluded canal, and that therefore the drum is behaving differently in the two situations even though the pressure in the cavity is the same.

Response Curve of the Ear

We have already intimated, in our discussion of the external ear, that characteristics of ear structures influence the transmission of acoustic energy at different frequencies. It is instructive to compare these effects over the frequency range with the shape of the sensitivity curve. Shaw's frequency response curve for each of the elements was shown in Fig. 3 beginning with the baffle effect of the head and ending at the eardrum. Already the shape of the auditory sensitivity curve, as shown in the Sivian and White curve, began to appear. We added the transfer function of the middle ear and the overall shape of the curve showed an even stronger resemblance, to the measured sensitivity curve (Zwislocki, 1975). There is still a discrepancy in the shape of the two curves. The greatest departure is at fairly low frequencies where measured sensitivity grows more rapidly with increasing frequency than the composite mechanical curve predicts. It may be that over this frequency range, where frequency following by nerve impulses is very good, the number of nerve spikes per unit time doubles with each increase of an octave even when level remains constant, and this could account for the difference in slope—3 dB/octave over this range.

The extreme low-frequency segment of the curve has now been measured with much better equipment than was available to Békésy. Because pure tones at extremely low frequencies are not easy to produce, Whittle et al. (1972) used a pressure chamber to expose their listeners to sinusoidal variations of pressure at frequencies from 50 Hz down to 3.15 Hz. Their measurements do not differ by more than a few dB from the dashed extrapolation of the MAP curve of Fig. 21. Yeowart et al. (1967) who made measurements over a similar frequency range, have pointed out that, even though the input signal is sinusoidal, at frequencies below about 15 Hz the sensation is no longer tonal.

From 15 Hz down to 5 Hz their subjects described it as "rough" or "popping". And from 5 Hz down to the lowest frequency they measured, which was 1.5 Hz, it sounded like "chugging" or "whooshing". It must be that at these slow rates of movement, some small amount of fluid is forced back and forth all along the cochlea and some flows through the helicotrema during each cycle.

The point along this low frequency segment that is the end of the *tonal* range of hearing is not easily determined. We will discuss this question further when we explore the perception of the pitch of tones.

At the high end of the frequency range it is again difficult to decide what is the exact frequency limit of the ear. As we noted in discussing the mechanical behavior of the cochlea each point on the basilar membrane responds best to a restricted range of frequencies. As the input frequency moves above this range of best frequencies for any given point, the amplitude of that point goes down extremely rapidly as frequency increases (see the shape of the amplitude envelope in Fig. 10). The most basalward segment of the membrane must be most responsive to some frequency that should be identified as the top of the auditory range. Yet although sensitivity drops sharply above about 12 kHz (Northern et al., 1972; Rice et al., 1969), auditory sensation can be elicited with input frequencies as high as 100 kHz. At such high frequencies the stimulus is more easily introduced by bone conduction rather than air conduction, but the resulting pitch sensation indicates that the same thing is happening to the extreme basal end as happens when it is driven around 15—20 kHz. Corso and Levine (1965) demonstrated the truth of this latter statement by showing that subjects match the pitch of different tones in the range of 50 to 100 kHz to the pitch of about 17 kHz.

This pitch response to frequencies apparently well above the characteristic frequency of the "end" of the membrane is puzzling. Over the rest of the length of the basilar membrane, the amplitude of response of a segment responding best to a particular frequency drops at rates of 100 dB/octave or better. Fortunately, it need be of only passing interest. The oft-repeated statement that the effective frequency range of human hearing is from 20 Hz to 20 kHz is still a reasonable assessment, even though we now know more about how quasi-auditory behavior at both ends makes the exact range more difficult to establish.

We have spoken of the lowermost curves of Fig. 21 as representing the absolute sensitivity of the ear. In the older literature on audition one is likely to see an emphasis on the difference between absolute threshold and relative thresholds. First of all, the supposition was that the beginning of auditory sensation is a step-like phenomenon and then by implication that the measuring of threshold in the presence of ambient noise is a fundamentally different operation than measuring its absolute (quiet) threshold.

Now there is good evidence that, at least over part of the frequency range, inherent physiological noise is the determiner of the minimum audibility curve that we measure, and furthermore that since all measured units of the auditory nerve exhibit spontaneous random firing rates in the absence of a signal, these two processes—the measurement of absolute sensitivity and the detection of a signal in the presence of noise are substantially the same. Neither is properly regarded as a "threshold" phenomenon. The term is still widely applied, but it should be recognized as a misnomer.

Another consequence of this signal-in-noise aspect of minimum audibility is that binaural thresholds will differ from monaural since the noise in the two ears will not be identical. We will hold further discussion of this aspect until we look at binaural phenomena.

The tonal signals used in establishing the curves in Fig. 21 have been a half second or longer in duration. If shorter tones are used, a critical duration is reached below which amplitude must be increased to keep the tone detectable. In general, below this critical duration, which turns out to be about 200 msec, the intensity of the tone (proportional to amplitude squared) must be doubled when the duration is halved. In other words, $I_{th} \times D = C$, where I_{th} is the intensity to keep the sound just detectable (at threshold) as duration changes. The system is behaving as though it uses an integrator with a time constant of about 200 msec in detecting the presence of short signals, and thus behaves as the analog of an energy detector. It is, of course, an oversimplification, since the behavior persists when the detection is binaural with changing interaural conditions, but it is a useful way to understand and remember the behavior of the ear in detecting short signals. A similar mechanism seems to operate in mediating the loudness of short signals *above* threshold. Loudness measurement is somewhat more variable than detection, so the function is not so well established for stronger signals.

The curves we have discussed, mostly from Fig. 21, are derived with a few listeners very carefully selected and trained and the listening environment well isolated and highly absorbent. The statistical nature of minimum audibility data under more representative listening conditions will be more thoroughly treated when we discuss the measurement of hearing loss.

Before leaving the discussion of the sensitivity curve, we should note that the most important set of auditory signals, the sounds of speech, nestle felicitously in the trough of the sensitivity curve when speech is very faint. We might postulate that at the end of a long evolutionary development this must be true for any species that depends, for survival, on communication with its own kind. For mankind there may have been a long interplay of evolutionary and more obvious short-term adaptive responses that have brought this about, but whatever the causes we seem to have reached a fortunate congruence of production and reception of the sounds of communication.

By contrast, sensitivity for high frequency, above 20 kHz, increased steadily in the phyletic development leading to Man (Masterton *et al.*, 1969). Among the mammals, only Man and the apes have relatively poor sensitivity above about 20 kHz. Whether this is related to an upright head and wideset ears and is therefore tied to the importance of sound localization is now difficult to determine.

7 Frequency Analysis: Pitch

Since nearly all the sounds useful to the auditory system are complex sounds, the ability of the system to separate these sounds into their separate frequency constituents is one of its most important attributes. Immediately, however, we face a dilemma. Any spectrum analyzer that accomplishes fine frequency resolution will be correspondingly slow in following temporal changes in the signal. We sometimes encounter this accidentally in a loudspeaker system. If the speaker has any sort of resonant peak in the range of interest, signals in that part of the frequency range will be smeared in time—we are apt to say it loses clarity. The sharper the peak the worse it muddles the time pattern at that frequency.

It looks as though the auditory system attempts a solution to this problem by having not one analyzer but several. Out at the cochlea, where ideally both options would be kept open, a dual function looks quite likely. If we look closely at the modern revision of the frequency response of a segment of the cochlear partition, as shown in Fig. 23, it appears that the fiber associated with this segment may contribute to fine frequency analysis when some component of the signal lies near the characteristic frequency—the peak of the curve—but contribute to a different aspect of analysis when the signal lies in the parts of the spectrum further from this best frequency. The entire cochlea may be contributing, at the same time, outputs from a narrow filter for optimum frequency separation and outputs from a fairly broad low-pass filter that preserves more of the timing information at the expense of fine frequency resolution. This possibility is supported by some experiments of Kiang and Moxon (1974) indicating that low frequency information is available in the tails of the tuning curves of fibers with high characteristic frequency. From a glance back at Fig. 17 it is also evident that some fibers with high characteristic frequency respond over a wide frequency range when the signals are of moderate level.

These examples are relevant, but the larger principle for our present discussion is the fact that the auditory system is a much more facile and

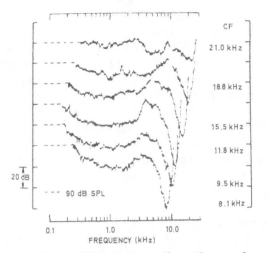

Fig. 23. The response area of several high-frequency fibers. These are from the auditory nerve of the cat. The curve for each fiber shows, for each frequency, the lowest level that evoked a discernible response from the fiber (see Fig. 16). Vertical placement of the curves is arbitrary; the dashed line indicates a test-signal SPL of 90 dB, and the range is indicated at the right in 20 dB increments. Also shown on the right is the characteristic frequency of each fiber plotted. (From Kiang and Moxon, 1974)

complex spectrum analyzer than we are apt to envision when we attempt to concentrate on a single aspect—in this instance, the pitch response.

Because of this complexity of auditory spectral analysis, we need to be aware that the perceptual output from various spectral analyses will take different forms. We might, for the sake of explanatory convenience, divide these many responses into two classes: pitch responses and sound quality responses. Even this dichotomy must be adopted only tentatively because ambiguity develops between these two for certain signals. Particularly for unfamiliar sounds, when certain changes are made in the spectrum, some listeners may judge that the pitch has changed and others insist it was a change in sound quality.

The Nature of Pitch

Pitch is conveniently defined as the perceptual response to frequency placement or frequency pattern of auditory signals. Although for many simple signals it varies monotonically with frequency it is most confusing to use it as a direct synonym, even where the relation is very close. It should not be used to refer to the physical measure.

Even for the simplest of tones, single-frequency sinusoids of fairly long duration, we have two different scales relating pitch to frequency. One of these is familiar to most of us. It derives from the musical scale and it treats all logarithmically equal frequency differences as equal pitch differences. Any semitone difference in the scale of a keyboard instrument (equal-tempered scale) is taken (uncritically, at least) to be the same subjective size as another semitone. Thus, at least in Western cultures, over the entire range of musical pitches a frequency ratio of 1.059 : 1, the ratio for a semitone difference, is treated as a constant difference in pitch. This frequency ratio derives from dividing the octave (a frequency ratio of 2 : 1) into twelve equal logarithmic steps ($2^{1/12} \simeq 1.059$). Even here, however, the influence of listening context on the response of the auditory system must be taken into account. Most people can reproduce the major scale readily, but it usually takes some thought for non-musicians to say which scale steps are semitones and which are full tones. On casual listening, diatonic scale steps are equal. But in a succession of semitones, a chromatic run, successive intervals seem the same size to most listeners.

But does this equal-ratio division of the frequency range represent the basic relation between frequency and perceptual response, or is it a convenient compromise to make musical scales and instruments more mathematically tractable? Long ago, Stevens (1937) set out to derive from formal listening experiments some systematic structuring of the relation between pitch distances and frequency changes, minimally influenced by the listeners' already-established musical conditioning. Subjects were required to set frequency control dials until a pitch sounded, say, half as high as a standard, or subjects were asked to create, in another part of the frequency domain, a pitch distance that matched one already set—all this without regard to musical reference. The scale that emerges from such operations departs considerably from the semitone structure described above, as can be seen in Fig. 24. These data are from Stevens and Volkmann (1940), and the scale was named the mel scale from the word melody. This might seem paradoxical considering that the musical scale on this same graph would be a straight line. Since distances along the basilar membrane appear to be equal for equal ratio of best frequency at any 2 points

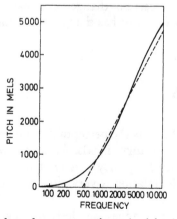

Fig. 24. The relation of pitch to frequency as determined by judgment of tonal distances. The dashed line indicates equal numbers of mels per octave. In the frequency range most frequently used for vocal melody the mel curve departs most from a straight line. (From Stevens *et al.*, 1937)

(Greenwood, 1962; Siebert, 1962), perhaps we should not be too strongly influenced by the ends of the mel scale where the two scales disagree most. Over most of the musical pitch range, namely about 200 Hz to 4000 Hz the departure from straight line is not so drastic.

What should be remembered is that the mel scale was built on judgments of the pitch-frequency relation for pure tones rather than complex tones, and definitely outside a musical context. This has a definite bearing on how generally the mel scale should be taken to be *the* scale of pitch. Other listening contexts also have strong effects, and the uncritical extrapolation of the use of the mel scale to all auditory judgments related to frequency, for instance the pitch of one partial of a complex tone, or the effect of any frequency-related change not involving a specific judgment of pitch is not automatically appropriate. Any scale is defined by the operations used to derive it. Particularly in subjective scaling, the more these operations depart from our usual experiences with the attribute, the greater the likelihood that the scale will not be universally applicable to that attribute.

Pitch Change

Pitch scales suggest that changes in the frequency of a sinusoidal tone seem to be paralleled by changes in position along a perceptual continuum. This is the most rudimentary analysis—different frequencies lead to different pitches. One might next ask how fine are the steps along this subjective dimension. It is a question possibly as old as music itself, but it required relatively modern equipment to fashion a fairly complete answer. Shower and Biddulph (1931) at the Bell Telephone Laboratories presented listeners with tones that stayed at a single frequency for a time then moved smoothly to a second frequency at a progressively smaller distance, and they ascertained at how small a difference their listeners could tell the frequency had changed. This is by definition the smallest frequency change that leads to a reliable judgment of pitch change—the just noticeable difference (jnd) in frequency.

This relative jnd ($\Delta f/f$) has been investigated for both frequency and intensity in audition and for a number of other sensory reactions. It is sometimes known as the Weber fraction because back in 1834 Weber proposed that the just discernible change in a physical correlate of a sensory dimension was a constant fraction of the value of the dimension at the point of measurement. The Shower and Biddulph results are shown in Fig. 25. It is apparent that with the method they used the relative amount of frequency change ($\Delta f/f$) decreases drastically at low frequencies and tends to level off for frequencies above 1 kHz. It is also apparent that the size of this smallest discernible difference in frequency changes with the level of the tone. Each curve in Fig. 25 is for a different Sensation Level, *i.e.*, a different number of decibels above threshold.

This set of curves has been the standard for the jnd in frequency for many years. Other less extensive studies have contributed other estimates and have also demonstrated that using a different method than the slowly varying tones

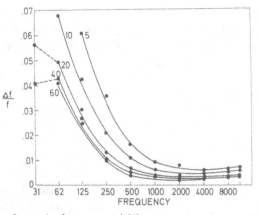

Fig. 25. The relative change in frequency ($\Delta f/f$) necessary to hear a change in pitch. This is the amount of change necessary when the tone changes slowly and continuously. Numbers at the top left of each curve denote the sensation level of the tone. (From Shower and Biddulph, 1931)

of Shower and Biddulph one gets a different estimate of the jnd. Recently Wier, Jestead and Green (1977) did a comparable exploration of jnd in frequency using a pair of sinusoidal bursts about a half second in duration. Each time a pair of tones was presented the subject was required to say whether the first or second tone was the higher of the two. After each trial he was told whether he was correct. A series of such trials begins with a frequency difference large enough to be discriminated, and this difference is decreased whenever the subject gets two consecutive pairs correct, and increased after every incorrect pair (Levitt, 1971). This allows the experimenter to estimate the 71 % correct point. The results of this study are shown in Fig. 26 along

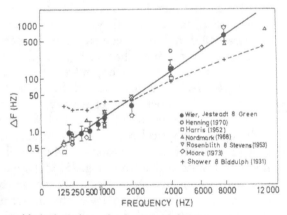

Fig. 26. The heavy black dots show the frequency difference necessary to hear a change in pitch when two separate tones are presented at a moderate level (40 dB SL). The data for other experimenters is identified. It is also for tones at about the same level. The straight line is the line of best fit to the black dots. Note that the Shower and Biddulph data—for tones that glided slowly up or down in frequency—does not fit with other data. The fact that the +'s make nearly a horizontal line could mean that Δf is constant below 1 kHz (see text). (From Wier et al., 1977)

with earlier measurements by others. Rather than showing $\Delta f/f$, this portrayal shows the frequency difference Δf along the ordinate.

Looking at the Shower and Biddulph results compared to others, it is apparent that changing the frequency gradually from one value to the others yields a different jnd than the other methods. Which is the correct one? Obviously it depends on the use one wishes to make of the information. If we assume these results can be generalized to apply to perceiving the mis-tuning of musical notes, then listening to discrete tones comes closer to the same operation. If we ask instead about the system's ability to discern slight changes in speed of some rotating device that produces a tone then the Shower and Biddulph method is more appropriate.

In Fig. 26 can be seen support for an easy rule of thumb for the necessary frequency change to make a just noticeable difference in pitch. Looking at the $+$'s of the Shower and Biddulph data it appears that at frequencies up to about 1 kHz a constant Δf of about 3 Hz is required, whereas at higher frequencies a constant $\Delta f/f$ of about 0.003 is a reasonable estimate. This was adopted as a reasonable rule of thumb following the Shower and Biddulph data. It has some additional appeal because the evidence from neurophysiology indicates that, early in the auditory system, neural firings tend to bunch at particular points in the cycle, so that a cycle-counting mechanism would be feasible. The higher the frequency the more difficult it is to maintain this frequency-locked firing pattern, so it could well be that a different mechanism is better for registering fine pitch differences at high frequencies.

Unfortunately for this simple rule of thumb, there is very little support from the other data in Fig. 26 for a Δf that remains constant over much of the frequency range.

Sometimes $\Delta f/f$ is preferred over just the frequency difference because it can be easily interpreted as a fraction of musical semitones. In addition to the use of semitones as the twelfth root of 2, very fine differences in frequency can be designated in musical cents, one cent being the 1200th root of 2 or 1/100 of a semitone. Tables of cent values are not common, but using a table of common logs $\Delta f/f$ values can be transformed to fractions of a musical semitone by noting that

$$\text{Semitone difference} = 12 \log_2\left(1 + \frac{\Delta f}{f}\right)$$

$$= (12)(3.32) \log_{10}\left(1 + \frac{\Delta f}{f}\right)$$

$$\approx 40 \log_{10}\left(1 + \frac{\Delta f}{f}\right) \qquad (\log_{10} X = 3.32 \log_2 X)$$

Multiplying this figure by 100 gives the difference between the two frequencies in cents.

The value 1.003 from the old rule of thumb amounts to only 5 cents or 1/20 of a semitone. In the range of good pitch discrimination, the line of best fit to most of the data in Fig. 26 stays close to 1.002. This is much finer frequency discrimination than is called for in normal listening and probably even for musical performance. It is of at least passing interest in this regard that a number of experimenters on jnd in frequency have noted that subjects with greatest musical experience are not necessarily those with best performance on this laboratory task.

No matter which experimenter's results we choose from Fig. 26 it is clear that the auditory system can tell when two successively presented pure tones differ only very slightly in frequency. As a matter of incidental interest, in the middle range (around 1 kHz) there are about 500 rows of hair cells per octave. The best pitch discriminators under ideal conditions can hear a change of about 2 cents, so we must conclude that something in the system is detecting a change when the maximum on the membrane has shifted by just about the spacing of adjacent hair cells. There is little question that even for this fairly straight-forward task considerable post-cochlear processing is required.

The measurements shown in Fig. 26 were taken on tones of fairly long duration. The only data shown there for tones shorter than half a second are taken from Moore (1973). These are for tones lasting 200 msec. Actually Moore presented his subjects with much shorter tones also, down to as short as 6.25 msec. Even for these very short tones, a good subject can hear frequency differences of less than 1 % (about a fifth of a semitone) for frequencies of 1 kHz to 4 kHz, and less than 2 % for 500 Hz. For durations between 6.25 and 100 msec performance improves until at durations of 100 msec the results are nearly the same as those shown in Fig. 26. A number of other studies on frequency discrimination for short tones are essentially in agreement with this result (Chih-an and Chistovich, 1960; Sekey, 1963; Cardozo, 1962).

Thus the situation seems to be that shorter and shorter tone bursts still continue to elicit an identifiable pitch response, even though the variability, as indicated by the jnd, gets progressively larger with decreasing duration. One convenient end point would be a tone burst consisting of a single cycle. Does it still elicit a consistent pitch response? Part of the problem in answering that question is producing such waveforms acoustically. Jenkins-Lee (1971) succeeded in doing so with a special ion-cloud transducer for faithfully producing single-sinusoid acoustic pressure changes. His subjects could tell correctly 75 % of the time which was the higher frequency of a pair of such short signals when they differed in frequency, or period, by 10 %. This is roughly two musical semitones (one scale step), so precision of frequency discrimination has decayed considerably compared to that for long tone bursts.

Perhaps the reason for this decay in precision of the pitch-discrimination response is attributable to the fact that as the tone burst is made shorter its spectrum grows correspondingly wider. Fig. 27 shows the spectrum of the single-cycle bursts used by Jenkins-Lee. Obviously, the pattern on the basilar membrane in addition to being fleeting in time is considerably spread. The complex auditory analyzer, faced with the task of differentiating two such spectrally-smeared signals may also choose not to compare spectral patterns but to make use of the difference in time period of the two waveforms. Frequency measurement, we recall, can also be accomplished by measuring the period of a waveform.

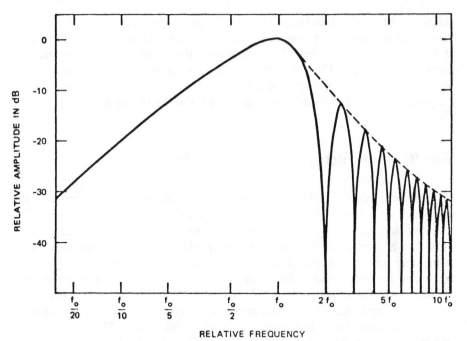

Fig. 27. The spectrum of a single cycle of a sinusoid. Note that the frequency scale is logarithmic to suggest roughly its contribution to the excitation pattern in the cochlea. That pattern must be both short and widespread. If the number of cycles is increased, the width of the center peak decreases

There is already some evidence that the auditory system derives a pitch from the spacing of the beginning and end of a single period.

A study by McClellan and Small (1967) employed signals of the same length as those of Jenkins-Lee, but an entirely different waveform. They presented a single signal consisting of two sharp pulses and ascertained whether the pitch of that signal corresponded to the period between the two pulses. They did so by asking subjects (music students) to match the pitch of the pulse pair to the pitch of a pure tone. The frequencies set by the subjects when they indicated the two signals (sinusoid and pulse pair) were matched in pitch cluster closely enough to indicate the pulse pair has a definite pitch. In the best range, around 400—500 Hz, most errors are within a semitone of the modal frequency—not too different from the uncertainty of judging Jenkins-Lee's single-period sinusoids—and the modal frequency of the matching sinusoids did have nearly the period of the pulse-pair spacing. This pitch has been called "time separation pitch" and can be taken as one kind of evidence for the auditory system's use of time period information, rather than some correlate of spectral placement, in making judgments of pitch.

All these time-pattern oriented pitch responses come conveniently under the rubric "periodicity pitch", whereas spectral cues are taken to contribute to "place pitch". We will look at both more broadly when we discuss the pitch of complex tones. One point to be remembered from this discussion of the pitch of short signals is that although pitch judgements show greater uncertainty, *i.e.*, the jnd in frequency gets larger as the signals get shorter, even very short signals have a reasonably definite pitch. There has been a seemingly attractive notion that there is a duration "threshold" for the sensation of pitch (Doughty and Garner, 1947, cited extensively since), but it has little or no experimental support. Neither does it fit with the use of such musical pitches as the sound of wood blocks or rapidly damped tympani notes.

Simultaneous Pitches

Our analysis thus far has dealt with pitch-difference judgment for two successively presented signals. If we still restrict our interest to sinusoidal tones it is instructive to ask how close in frequency two simultaneously-present tones can be and still elicit two separate pitches. Most of us remember from elementary physics of sound that when two pure tones of nearly the same frequency are present in a linear device they sum linearly from moment to moment and the result is a signal of essentially sinusoidal waveform that changes in amplitude from a minimum when the two tones are in opposite phase to a maximum when they are in the same phase. These maxima (or minima) have the spacing of the frequency difference of the two tones, so we say the two tones "beat" at a rate corresponding to their frequency difference in Hertz. As this frequency difference increases and the fluctuation becomes more rapid, the auditory impression changes from that of a beating tone to a rough tone instead. This transition is not abrupt, but takes place gradually between about 6 or 7 beats per second, about the rate of the frequency or amplitude vibrato of musical sounds, and 12—15 physical beats per second. At this latter frequency separation, the perceived tone is definitely rough.

As the separation is increased further, considerable perceptual uncertainty sets in, as indicated by the shaded area in Fig. 28. This is a portrayal by Plomp of the area within which there is some, but not unanimous, agreement that two simultaneous tones give rise to two pitches if they are separated as shown on the ordinate and in the frequency region shown by the abscissa. As an example, for two tones in the neighborhood of 200 Hz, some listeners have reported two pitches when the two tones are separated by only 10 Hz, but others not until the tones are 100 Hz apart.

For separations of 30 Hz and less, the single pitch that is heard is a pitch between the pitches that would be elicited by the two tones heard separately. This is the pitch of the intertone. It is determined by matching it to another pure tone. It may be audible when the separation is even greater (Nordmark, 1978). Actually, because this separation appears related to the consonance of musical sounds most experimenters have been interested in the roughness of the tone in this region rather than in its pitch.

The other phenomenon of interest that occurs at some frequency separation of the two tones is that the roughness gives way to, or else is accompanied by, a low pitch associated with the difference in frequency between the two tones.

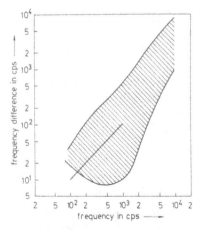

Fig. 28. The area of uncertainty regarding the hearing of two separate pitches when two pure tones are present. For two-tone combinations that lie below the shaded area only a single (rough) tone is heard. For combinations that lie above the area listeners definitely hear two separate pitches. The main point conveyed by the graph is that there is great disagreement about when two pure tones give rise to two pitches. The straight line indicates a separation of one full musical tone. With that signal, most music students can easily identify both pitches. (From Plomp, 1964a)

This can come about in two ways. One way stems from the periodic nature of the envelope of the waveform of two simultaneous tones whenever the separation in frequency is sufficiently smaller than the frequency of the two tones. Fig. 29 shows the appearance of a beat-like or modulated waveform. Referring back to our slowly beating waveform, it is apparent that the spacing of the envelope maxima will be the period of the difference frequency between the two tones. Since the probability of neural units firing is directly related to the amplitude of the signal, we have a periodic neural time pattern at the frequency of the difference. Much evidence now exists that such a periodic time pattern in the tonal frequency range leads to the perception of a pitch in the same range as a pure tone that has that same period. This kind of pitch is much more prominent when there are several tones with that same spacing, as is the case with harmonic partials of many complex tones.

The other way in which the same pitch might arise relates to the fact that if the mechanism responding to the two simultaneous tones has some non-

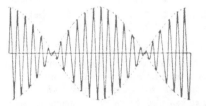

Fig. 29. Waveform of the mixture of two tones when the frequency difference is much smaller than their average frequency. The dotted line traces what is usually referred to as the envelope

linearity in its response, there will actually be some energy at the difference frequency. The difference between these two sources of the pitch response must be clear. In one instance the pitch is arising from neural fibers at the *place* of the harmonics, *but firing at the rate of the envelope or frequency difference.* In the other case, there is actually a sinusoidal component added at the frequency of the difference, and presumably it has its effect by exciting the cochlea at the point that is resonant to the frequency of the difference.

For the moment let us follow our two simultaneous tones as they are separated even further, at which point their two separate pitches can be heard. When this occurs, the roughness tends to disappear (Plomp, 1966). It seems the spectrum analysis done by the auditory system has now clearly separated the two tones. It is as though in the laboratory we had set an adjustable filter such that if we centered it on the first tone there would be no interference from the second, and vice versa. The separation at which this occurs seems to have a general auditory significance, as we shall see when we discuss other aspects of frequency resolution. We say the tones are separated by a critical bandwidth.

Pitch of Complex Tones

Pure tones, we recognize, are not the usual signal for the auditory system. A few everyday sounds are nearly single frequency—the flute or piccolo tone, some organ tones, some whistle tones. Most tones used in the laboratory have been pure tones, and one reason to be interested in their single un-ambiguous pitch is their use for matching the pitch of complex sounds.

On superficial inspection, the pitch of complex tones appears to present no particular problems. If we look for too close a parallel with pure tones and recall that a steady-state complex tone can be viewed as a sum of harmonically related pure tones, the possibility of multiple pitches might arise. However, when an orchestra tunes to the A-440 of, say, the oboe, the players all tune their instruments to A-440—or an octave below—not to one of the other notes suggested by its harmonic partials[2] or overtones (see Fig. 31). There is, in practice at least, no equivocation about the pitch of a musical complex tone.

If we try to be a bit more analytical and assign the task of matching a sinusoid, with energy at just one point in the spectrum, to a complex tone, the match will nearly always be made to the fundamental. Actually, a long time before such a maneuver was possible, *i.e.,* before the day of wide-range

---

[2] If the reader remembers, from elementary physics of sound, that periodic complex tones can be described as the sum of harmonically related sinusoidal tones, the distinction in usage of partials and harmonics should be easy to keep in mind. Any one of the sinusoidal tones that could be separated out from the complex waveform is referred to as a partial. If the complex tone is periodic it can also be called a harmonic partial, or harmonic. Sometimes we build tonal complexes from sinusoidal components that do not belong in the harmonic series. These are referred to as partials or inharmonic partials depending on whether the text has made clear which it is.

pure tone oscillators, conventional wisdom had it that the pitch of a complex tone was determined by the fundamental. With the discovery that filtering out the fundamental, as happens for example to the speech of the male voice heard over the telephone, does not change the perceived pitch, some revision of this explanation was required.

We would find, if we traced the history of pitch perception of complex tones more accurately, that the idea that the energy at the fundamental was the sole determiner of the pitch of the tone had been challenged long before the problem was posed by the restricted band of the telephone. Seebeck, back in 1841, created complex tones through the use of rotating discs with spaced air holes for creating a train of pulses (a type of air siren). By asymmetric placing of the holes he could generate tones with very little energy at the fundamental frequency. He championed the view that it was the periodicity of a regular pattern that was perceived as the pitch. Ohm, generator of Ohm's acoustic law, argued instead that even for a tone with no energy at the fundamental, the ear possessed sufficient nonlinearity that it generated a difference tone between adjacent harmonics, and this difference tone re-introduced energy at the fundamental frequency. What Ohm described is true, but Schouten showed some considerable time later (1940) that if the re-introduced fundamental energy is cancelled the pitch of the complex tone remains the same. He called this remaining pitch the residue. The analytical listener can hear, as Schouten did, both these pitches by alternately removing and restoring the energy at the fundamental. At low frequencies the contrast between the two is that the fundamental energy has the sound of a hum, whereas the residue is more of a pulse train or buzz-like sound.

But during the time of Seebeck and Ohm this was not known, and it happened that Helmholtz threw his considerable weight behind the Ohm side of the argument. Only gradually has the idea gained credence that periodic patterns of nerve firing may themselves be strong clues in the perception of pitch. Possibly the most persuasive demonstration of this kind of periodicity pitch was presented by Davis and his cohorts (1951). They took a fairly narrow filter tuned to around 2000 Hz and pulsed it at a rate of 150 pulses per second. They asked listeners to match the pitch of the resulting sound to a pure tone. All listeners reported the pitch as a buzz, and only a few matched the sinusoid to the 2000 Hz frequency rather than to the 150/sec pulsing rate. What makes this example so nearly appropriate is that it has the rudiments of a musical instrument. Most instruments consist at least partly of one or more resonances excited by a driving source of lower frequency than that of the resonance. Predictably, when the pulsing frequency and the resonant (filter) frequency were moved independently in the Davis *et al.* example, listeners recognized that the filter placement determined the quality of the sound whereas the pulsing rate was more closely related to the pitch. In general, this is an acceptable view of difference between pitch and quality of complex tones, namely that their pitch frequently corresponds to the lowest frequency, the quality, or timbre, of the tone corresponds to the shape of the spectrum or the characteristic spectral peaks. We have already seen, however, that complex tone pitch is not always that simple.

Some of the confusion about what determines fundamental pitch was cleared by an experiment of Flanagan and Guttman (1960). They chose the waveforms of Fig. 30 to pit pulse rate against fundamental frequency in determining pitch. Note that waveform A and B can have the same number of pulses per second, but the spectrum of A would then have a fundamental frequency an octave lower. When subjects are given control of the frequency of A and asked to match it to the pitch of B they match pulse for pulse at frequencies below 125 pulses per second in spite of the octave difference in fundamental. Above about 200 pulses per second matches were made to fundamental frequency in spite of differences in pulse rate. For this set of signals at least, timing information predominates in determining the pitch only at low frequencies.

There is other, less easily described, evidence that timing information contributes to determining the pitch of complex tones. So, of course, does spectral information either in the form of place of fundamental or pattern of spacing of harmonics. Considering the complexity of auditory processing and the variety of pitch perceptions, there seems little purpose in choosing one to the exclusion of the other. A sufficiently versatile and adaptive sensory system should make use of whatever clues yield satisfactory information about events of interest in the environment, and will probably be characterized by redundancy of information rather than parsimony. We have ample reason to believe both kinds of information are available to the auditory processor.

A number of clever maneuvers have been employed in the laboratory to explicate the details of the pitch perceiving mechanism. Signals with only a selected number of high-numbered partials can be created through amplitude modulation. If, for instance, one listens to a tone consisting of energy at 1800, 2000 and 2200 Hz, the pitch corresponding to that of a 200 Hz tone is present, but not strong. As other partials that are multiples of 200 are added, the strength of the low pitch increases. This can be interpreted to mean that for a tone with many partials, envelope maxima at the 200/sec rate are present at many points in the cochlea and contribute to a dominant pitch of the fundamental.

The tone of 1800, 2000 and 2200 Hz has usually been created by multiplying a 2000 Hz carrier by a 200 Hz modulator and then re-introducing the carrier:

$$f(t) = \sin (2_\pi) (2000) \, t \, [1 + \sin (2_\pi) (200) \, t].$$

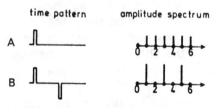

Fig. 30. Two waveforms which have the same fundamental frequency but a different number of pulses per fundamental period. Note that spacing of the partials also differs—the lower waveform has no energy in the even-numbered partials.
(From Flanagan and Guttman, 1960)

Accomplishing this in the laboratory means leading the output of the 2000 Hz oscillator and the separate 200 Hz oscillator to the inputs of a multiplier; to satisfy the first term inside the brackets, a separate output from the carrier (2000 Hz) oscillator is added to the output of the multiplier. If we shift this part (the re-introduced carrier) by 90° before adding it back in, the resulting waveform would yield the same amplitude spectrum, but has practically no envelope variation. It looks more like a frequency-modulated wave than an amplitude-modulated one. It also has a very weak low pitch, confirming that for this signal the regular amplitude variation at 200/sec contributes to the perception of the "fundamental".

In our example, the 2000 Hz carrier and the 200 Hz modulator were chosen so that the resulting partials would be integer multiples of 200. If we move the carrier frequency to 2050 Hz, the waveform shows the maxima and minima at a spacing of 200/sec (though the peaks inside the envelope no longer have that exact spacing) and the low frequency pitch gets much weaker and somewhat ambiguous, to judge from the reports of various listeners and experimenters (Wightman, 1973 a). The pitch match most frequently offered in this instance is 205 Hz, but it is much more difficult to hear than the clear, salient pitch of a conventional musical tone.

Before chasing these elusive aspects of pitch any further, we should remember that in our discussion of the pitch behavior of two simultaneously-present sinusoids we saw that a listener could, with some exceptions, hear two separate pitches when the tones reached the spacing of a critical bandwidth. We shall see later, in describing the experiments that established the notion of a critical bandwidth for much of auditory processing, that the critical width corresponds to a ratio of ≈ 1.2 between upper and lower frequency limits of the band. Thus if we present the ear with two tones whose frequency ratio is greater than 1.2, the listener should hear a pitch for each.

If this were unqualifiedly true, then when all the partials of a complex tone are present we might expect to hear at least the separate pitches of the first six or seven partials, which have ratios to each other of about 1.2 or greater. Instead these partials tend to fuse into one fundamental pitch. Presumably, these tones, being quite completely separated from each other by auditory filtering, are not beating with each other at the common fundamental rate. There is ample evidence that they lead to synchronous neural firing, and this in itself might be expected to yield a more fused perception than for tones not so simply related. Worth noting is the fact if the partials are not quite exact multiples of the fundamental, the pitch is still unitary.

For these tones with the complete series of partials present, this is not the entire story of the pitch response. Analytical listeners can hear separately the pitch of each of the first seven or eight partials, but the contention is they cannot separate out the higher partials. This has been interpreted as further evidence of the operation of the critical-band filter (Plomp, 1976).

This is a persuasive argument, but it must be qualified for two reasons: (1) The method of establishing this limit has been to present a separate single-frequency tone and ask whether it is also present in the complex tone. For any partial where the off-frequency sinusoid could be identified as not being the one in the series, the conclusion was that the partial at that frequency was being heard. The problem is that the first eight harmonic partials—or higher ones for that matter—make an easily identifiable series of notes as shown in Fig. 31 (the seventh being musically out of tune). The second partial is an octave above the first; the third partial a perfect fifth above that; the fourth partial is two octaves above the fundamental; the fifth partial is two octaves plus a major third above the first one, but easily identifiable as the middle note of the major chord (triad) built on the fundamental; the sixth partial is just an octave above the third partial; and so until we reach the seventh partial anyone with minimal experience in music could identify a pure tone as being, or not being, in the

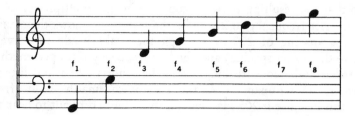

Fig. 31. One set of musical notes that follows the frequency sequence of the harmonic partials of a complex tone. The second harmonic partial, being twice the frequency of the first, is an octave above; the third harmonic partial is an octave plus a musical fifth (3/2) above the first, etc. We could, of course, start the sequence on any note. The lowest G could easily be tuned to 100 Hz (it is 98 Hz when A = 440) and then the frequencies of the others are automatically known

series simply from hearing the pitch of the fundamental. Nevertheless, the experiment comes out as auditory theory would predict. Ability to distinguish correct partial from mistuned sinusoid fails when the partials are no longer cleanly separable by a filter the width of the critical band. Considerable credence is added also by the report that for inharmonic partials the ability to hear components separately fails for about the same degree of frequency separation—namely about the width of the critical band (Soderquist, 1970). Independent corroboration comes from a technique for measuring frequency resolution called pulsation threshold measurement. This is described in the section on masking and the relevant results portrayed in Fig. 51. It is apparent that some aspect of frequency resolution changes at about the spacing of the 7th or 8th harmonic partial. (See p. 97.)

(2) There have been many reports of the selection of partials higher than the seventh or eighth, particularly by musical analytical listeners. Because the notes of familiar diatonic scale have simple frequency ratios simple scale passages and arpeggios can be performed by the successive selection of the appropriate harmonic partial. A slight change in amplitude or, as Schroeder has shown (1959), a sudden shift in phase can make a partial stand out for the auditory system. Such spectral melodies have made use of partials as high as the 20th to 24th. Thus the frequency-resolving capability of the auditory processor is not rigidly bounded by the width of the critical band.

Most of the time, in listening to complex tones, the system responds not with multiple pitches but by assigning a unitary definite pitch to the complex—so definite in fact, that, fine as we saw the discrimination of long pure tones to be, frequency discrimination for complex tones is even finer.

A number of modern theories have suggested the way in which a pattern is derived for the pitch of complex tones (Terhardt, 1974; Goldstein, 1973; Wightman, 1973 b; deBoer, 1977). For our purposes they do not differ. A composite view, which is reasonable for a versatile sensory channel is that pitch is probably arrived at by sensing the whole neural mosaic pattern contributed by the placement and the synchrony of the lower resolvable partials *and* the amplitude envelope from those partials too close together to be resolved by the critical band filter.

Our discussion of the pitch perceiving aspects of auditory frequency analysis has been primarily confined to steady-state, highly periodic tones. The system assigns a pitch, however, to much less periodic sounds than these. There are, even in music, less distinctly pitched sound than the sustained ones we usually associate with musical instruments.

But even more frequently we make a pitch oriented response to a variety of events in the environment. The filling of some containers is accompanied by a sound of rising pitch. Whether the wind is increasing or decreasing in velocity is often signalled by a rise or fall respectively in the pitch of the sound. The impact of, or on, a large object will in general be higher pitched than for a small one. A rise in vocal fundamental may signal excitement or emphasis; or the difference in rise or fall at the end of an utterance may help to differentiate between questions and declarations. Whether a number of useful devices are speeding up or slowing down can be discerned from a rise or fall in pitch. Even those "things that go bump in the night" can be more closely categorized depending on whether they make a low-pitched thud or a high-pitched snap.

Furthermore, many of the sounds processed by the auditory system —sounds in the environment or components in the sounds of speech—are not accurately described as sustained sounds. They are more nearly characterized by moment-to-moment changes in amplitude or frequency, and this means a departure from the discrete line spectrum of many laboratory-produced sounds. The most common classes are damped sinusoids, resulting from exciting some resonant body with an impulse, or bands of noise resulting from an aperiodic waveform transmitted through a poorly resonant air cavity like the vocal tract. This latter occurs for whispered speech, but also for the fricative sounds of regular speech production.

In the laboratory the pitch response to damped sinusoids has received very little attention. It's difficult to decide on the typical damping rates to use as prototypes in a laboratory study. Some applicable information on pitch response to such signals can be borrowed from the work on short tonal signals that we've already noted, since the spectra of short tone bursts and damped sinusoids are highly similar. The main difference between the two is a difference in the envelope of the waveform, and on this point a useful comparison comes from the work of Ronken (1971). Ronken explored pitch discrimination for 1 kHz signals with the envelope shapes shown in Fig. 32.

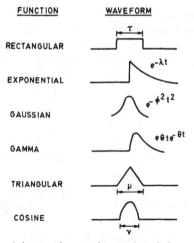

Fig. 32. The envelopes used by Ronken in his study of frequency discrimination. These patterns of rise and fall of tone amplitudes might easily occur in such natural sounds as speech, music or resonant environmental sounds. (From Ronken, 1971)

One can picture the signal waveforms more exactly by adding a symmetrical lower half to the envelope tracing and filling the space with sinusoids. He fashioned these signals so they would have equal spectrum widths and then compared the effect of these envelope shapes on pitch discrimination over a duration range from 2 to 32 msec. Ronken measured $\Delta f/f$ values and they are slightly higher than for the other studies with short square-envelope signals that we mentioned earlier. These differences, however, could readily be attributed to differences in the selection of listeners. The finding of interest within the study is that the smallest $\Delta f/f$ comes from the exponential envelope, most nearly resembling the shape of damped sinusoids. These are most like the transient sounds we encounter in everyday listening when some nearly untuned object is struck. The general principle is still upheld—that $\Delta f/f$ increases as durations are made shorter but there is no convincing evidence of a duration "threshold" for pitch discrimination. Pitch changes for rapidly-changing transient sounds are undoubtedly very useful to the system in identifying characteristics of sound sources in the environment.

The other class of quasi-periodic sounds, bands of noise, is easier to control in the laboratory. Pitch discrimination for bands of noise should not be expected to be as good as for pure tones since amplitude fluctuation will cause some interference even for fairly narrow bands. But even up to widths of 64 Hz shifts of about 1 % in the frequency position of the band can be correctly discerned (Michaels, 1957; Moore, 1973). The question arises whether shifts of that size in bands of noise are of anything but theoretical interest, since it's difficult to find examples in any of the useful distinctions that might be listed for auditory signals. Grosser shifts in the spectral position of noise bands are probably responded to as changes in sound quality rather than pitch, but we should remember that that division is arbitrary. We do not know how cleanly the auditory system separates the two in practice.

Loudness 8

In analyzing the sensitivity of the ear, we noted that sounds in the middle frequency range can vary in amplitude by a factor of a million to one and still be within the receptive capability of the ear. The response of the system to this large variation in amplitude or intensity is to register a difference in loudness. Thus loudness is the subjective parallel response to physical changes in intensity of sound much as pitch response parallels changes in frequency.

Even though the ear can operate over the tremendous range shown in Fig. 21, our preference is to have sounds lie in the middle of that range. One factor that narrows this total range of sounds is that many of the soft signals that can be heard in the quiet of the laboratory may well be masked out by the interfering sounds of everyday activities. Further, sounds that are just barely strong enough to be heard over interference are difficult to follow. We express this by saying we require a fairly good signal-to-noise ratio for comfortable listening.

In audition, what is meant by "signal-to-noise ratio"? In certain listening situations we can specify the energy in the desired sound and that in the unwanted sound in terms that make it useful to compute the signal to noise ratio by the decibel formula introduced previously

$$(S/N)_{dB} = 10 \log \frac{I_{signal}}{I_{noise}} = 20 \log \frac{P_{signal}}{P_{noise}}.$$

In a controlled laboratory situation this is what we use to specify the relations between signal and noise. Sometimes, even in the laboratory, neither signal nor noise can be measured with the precision or in the appropriate time relations to make this specification useful for auditory purposes. We frequently do not know how much of the noise spectrum is actually interfering with the signal or whether our measuring instrument averages the fluctuations in the noise in a way that corresponds with its auditory interference with the signal. In any situation where the signal can be changed by a controlled number of decibels (a gain control calibrated in dB, usually referred to as an attenuator) the solution is to set the level of the signal so that it can be detected some specified percentage of the time, usually 50 %, in a given level of the noise. This particular ratio of signal and noise—whatever its physical specifications—is defined as zero dB Sensation Level. If, without changing the noise, the level of the signal is increased by 10 dB, it is now at 10 dB Sensation Level (SL).

This concept of Sensation Level as the number of decibels above auditory threshold (however defined) is much more general than this example makes it seem. Even for readily specifiable signal and noise combinations it is sometimes useful to ignore sound pressure differences and emphasize the relative distance of two signals above their own auditory zero. Thus, Sensation Level of a signal is a frequently-used concept, and if carefully defined can be taken as the auditory signal-to-noise ratio.

Even at the same frequency, Sound Pressure Level and Sensation Level may not be simply related. In discussing auditory sensitivity, we noted that for tones of duration less than 200 msec amplitude had to be increased as duration shortened so that for equal detectability energy stayed constant. A similar situation holds for the loudness response to short tones. Comparing loudness for two signals (including tones or noises), both shorter than 80 msec, if one tone is only half as long as the other its intensity (or its pressure squared) must be doubled. Thus, up to a duration of 80 msec, energy must be equal for two signals to be equally loud (Scharf, 1978). For this same reason short explosive sounds may not seem as loud as their equivalent sound pressure amplitude would predict.

What must be remembered, however, is that even though we have set an auditory reference point in specifying Sensation Level, we have not converted the distance above that reference to loudness units. To do that, not just the zero point but the distances themselves would have to be compared and specified by a set of auditory judgments. This is akin to what we saw with the formulation of the mel scale for pitch. A loudness scale can be constructed even more easily, since here we don't have the problem of avoiding musical associations.

The basic principle in constructing a loudness scale is to use auditory judgments to determine relative distances between different levels of pure tones of the same frequency. Suppose, as with pitch, we start with a 1000 Hz tone at a median level of, perhaps 40 dB SL. We instruct the observer to set another tone twice as loud as this standard, and still another one half as loud. This can be continued toward both ends of the range and yields a number of trial points for a loudness function. The observer can also be asked to put a subjective-magnitude number to each of a set of tones at selected spaced intensities. These numbers can then be plotted as a loudness function. By using a number of such subjective comparisons of tones of different level, the loudness function shown in Fig. 33 was constructed. A 1 kHz tone at 40 dB SPL is assigned a loudness of 1 sone. Then it follows that the tone judged half as loud or assigned a magnitude number half as large has a loudness of $1/2$ sone, a tone judged twice as loud has loudness of 2 sones, etc. Given this curve, if we wish to compute the loudness of any pure tone knowing

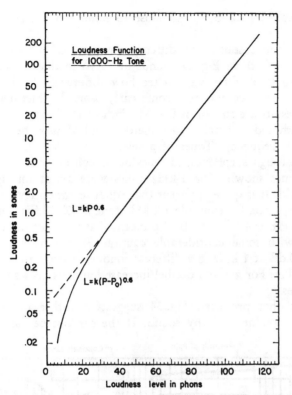

Fig. 33. Loudness as a function of Loudness Level. The value of k in the expression for loudness in sones *(L)* serves to fit the assigned loudness numbers to the units used for expressing the sound pressure *(P)*. (If P is measured in micropascals the value of k is 0.01.) To get a closer fit to the measured loudness near threshold the expression below the curve is used with Po equal to sound pressure at threshold. (From Scharf, 1978)

its sound pressure we can employ a convenient straight-line approximation curve

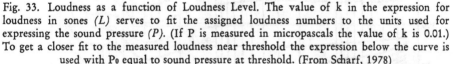

$$\text{Loudness in sones} = (p/p_{\text{ref}})^{0.6}$$

where p is the sound pressure of the tone in question and p_{ref} is the sound pressure of the standard 1-sone sound (40 dB SPL). It is also convenient to express the right hand side of the equation as $(I/I_0)^{0.3}$, remembering that the intensity ratio is the square of the pressure ratio. Either of these, then, shows that the subjective aspect, loudness, is related to the physical aspect, pressure or intensity, by a power law. The intensity expression is especially convenient for remembering a rule of thumb about loudness growth. Note that if we increase the intensity ratio by 10 we have multiplied the loudness by $10^{0.3}$ or 2. Thus every time we add 10 dB to a sound we double its loudness. This expression will be accurate for values above 40 dB SPL (1 sone) but will be progressively more inaccurate for lower levels. A closer approach, though not so convenient to remember, is (Scharf, 1978)

$$L_{\text{sones}} = 0.01 \, (p - 45)^{0.6}$$

since 45 μPascal is 7 dB SPL and close to minimum detectability level for 1 kHz.

But what about sounds of different frequencies? Obviously from our sensitivity curve back in Fig. 21 sounds of "zero loudness" are not of equal sound pressure level. One way to see how differently loudness behaves at different frequencies comes from some early work by Fletcher and Munson (1933). The results are shown in Fig. 34. Each of the heavy lines in the figure is actually anchored at 1 kHz, since Fletcher and Munson began with that as their standard frequency. Tones of a selected level at 1 kHz were matched in loudness, through earphones, to tones of enough other frequencies to draw the smooth lines shown. The 1 kHz tones were set at multiples of 10 dB above threshold. It is quite apparent that equal sensation level does not mean equal loudness, since, for example a 1 kHz tone at 70 dB SL is no louder than a tone of 100 Hz at 40 dB SL. It also means that we must use our power law of loudness with some considerable caution. If the scale is transitive an increase of 10 dB at 1 kHz is a different loudness change than an increase of 10 dB at 100 Hz. For a given decibel increase loudness grows most rapidly at low frequencies.

The work that produced Fig. 34 suggests a rather pragmatic way of measuring the loudness of any sound. If the ear can be used to match the

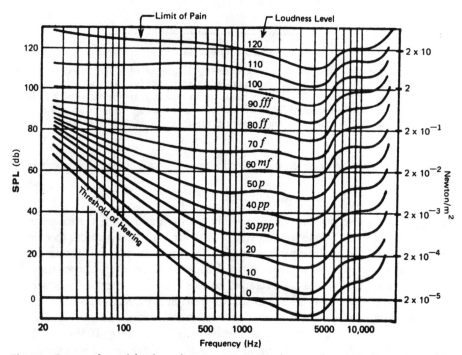

Fig. 34. Curves of equal loudness for pure tones. Numbers at the 1 kHz line are Loudness Levels in phons. Since all tones on a given contour are defined as having the same Loudness Level, a tone at a frequency far removed from 1 kHz may have quite a different phon value and SPL value. An approximation to musical designation of relative loudness is matched to the appropriate phon values. For some values of loudness corresponding to these phon values see Fig. 33. (From Fletcher and Munson, 1933)

loudness of any sound to that of a 1 kHz tone, then having a standard set of
values for each sound pressure level at 1 kHz permits assigning the value of
the matched 1 kHz tone to the sound in question. The new scale is called
Loudness Level and the numbers assigned are in phons, so that the basic definition reads that "The Loudness Level of a sound, in phons, is numerically equal
to the Sound Pressure Level of an equally loud tone of 1 kHz." Since the
threshold for 1 kHz is taken to be 7 dB SPL, adding 7 to each of the numbers
in the center of the graph of Fig. 34 gives the phons value of each tone on
that contour.

At this point we have an expression relating Loudness to Sound Pressure
or Intensity at 1 kHz and a table or graph showing how the loudness of 1 kHz
relates to that of other frequencies. What is needed is an expression relating
Loudness in sones to Loudness Level in phons. This has been derived
empirically from a large number of studies (Stevens, 1961, 1972) and a good
approximation is

$$\log L_{\text{sones}} = 0.03 \, P_{\text{phonc}} - 1.2.$$

In practice, the method is to measure the complex sound in octave or
$^1/_3$ octave segments. Sound Pressure Level is measured for each segment and
each of these values converted first to Loudness Level and then to Loudness
in sones. These loudness values can be combined into one total loudness for
the complex sound by another empirically-derived formula which takes
account of the fact that most of the loudness will be contributed by the band
with maximum loudness, and that the contribution of the other bands will
be influenced by how far apart they are, and therefore how much they interfere
with each other. The expression for combining $^1/_3$-octave bands is

$$L_{\text{total}} = L_{\text{max}} + 0.13 \sum (L_i - L_{\text{max}}).$$

Thus, the measurements of Fig. 34, or measurements like them, are useful in
arriving at loudness estimates for various complex sounds.

Whether the system is called upon to make judgments of minimal
difference in loudness is debatable, but the just noticeable difference in the
intensity of various sounds has at least been a matter of theoretical interest in
audition. It is possible to follow a procedure much like the studies of just
noticeable difference in frequency. The classic study in this area is one by
Riesz at the Bell Laboratories in 1928. He varied the intensity of his tones
by beating two tones with a frequency difference of 3 Hz. Changing the
intensity of the weaker tone changes the amplitude excursion of the beat. At
the point where the observer can just barely no longer discern that the tone is
beating, the difference between the maximum and minimum amplitude of the
beat is taken as the just noticeable difference.

So much of our work with the intensity dimension of the auditory system is
expressed in decibels that Riesz' work is best portrayed as in Fig. 35 with the
jnd expressed as ΔI in dB. Actually, this is shorthand notation for $10 \log$
$(I + \Delta I)/I$, but the shorter expression is useful because it indicates directly by
how many decibels a tone at a given level must change to lead to a perceptible
change in loudness.

The Riesz data have been taken to be the standard estimate of ΔI for years.

A number of smaller studies fairly recently have given essentially similar results for ΔI (Harris, 1963; McGill and Goldberg, 1968; Campbell and Lasky, 1967; Luce and Green, 1974). $\Delta I/I$, which should be a constant according to the original concept of Weber, changes considerably and apparently systematically over the intensity range, but particularly at low levels.

In 1977, Jestead, Wier, and Green did a very careful study over the same range of frequency and level as the Riesz study. The notable differences are that the tones compared were two 0.5-second bursts with a half second between rather than the slowly beating tone of the Riesz study, and the measuring method was the same as the adaptive sequence described earlier in the frequency discrimination study of Wier, Jestead and Green. ΔI in dB for the Jestead *et al.* study is described by the equation

$$10 \log \left[(I + \Delta I)/I \right] = 1.6 - \frac{\text{Sensation Level}}{70}$$

from which it is apparent that an increase of one dB will be a just noticeable change in intensity at a Sensation Level of about 40 dB.

This sort of simplicity for such an uncomplicated judgment is very comforting, but though it is an admirably careful study, it gives us no reason to discard the many other reasonable attempts to make the same measurement—only a few of them mentioned here. Recently Rabinowitz, Lim, Braida and Durlach (1976) summarized 15 studies on the jnd for intensity that all included measurements at the same frequency (1 kHz). They concluded that the response differed at low, middle and high intensities and fit a function of these to straight lines with different slopes.

Thus this seemingly straightforward response of judging whether the subjective strength of the simplest of auditory signals has changed perceptibly

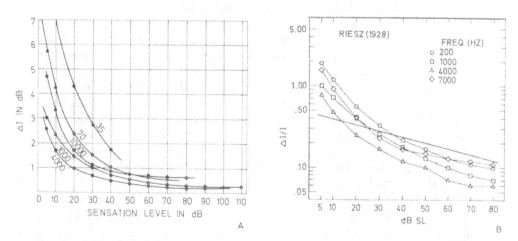

Fig. 35. *A* The decibel change necessary to make a just detectable change in the loudness of a tone. The necessary change not only differs for different frequencies (the numbers on the curves), but also depends on the Sensation Level of the tone. (From Riesz, 1928.) *B* Data for some selected frequencies of the Riesz study, plotted as the Weber fraction, $\Delta I/I$. The straight line is from the recent study of Jestead, Wier, and Green. (From Jestead *et al.*, 1977)

has caused all manner of disagreement among investigators. To add to the puzzle, the similar reaction to broadband noise has occasioned no such difficulty. Miller's measurement in 1947 indicated that the just perceptible change in the level of a broadband noise remains at 0.4 dB as the overall level of the noise varies from being just comfortably audible (about 20 dB SL) to 100 dB SL. This is a constant increase of about 5 %, and represents one of the few instances in audition of the Weber fraction remaining constant.

Why these rather sizeable differences in the estimates of the jnd for intensity? Which one is the right one? One answer to the first question is that this is not a highly practiced operation for the auditory system. True, the intensity dimension is an important one in audition and most signals of interest exhibit patterns of intensity variation. But as regards the perceptual response, there is a careful and important distinction to be made here. We may present the system with a pair of signals which differ only in intensity. If the time pattern of the signals and the listener's orientation are conducive to a perception of a change in loudness then it is useful to conclude that a loudness difference was perceived. When, however, the intensity change is so rapid or so linked to a different perception that the subject can only tell that he perceived a change and cannot identify it as a loudness change, it should not be labeled as such. Loudness, like pitch, is a subjectively determined dimension and should be labeled according to the listener's identification of the dimension—not the experimenter's knowledge of what physical change was made.

It is difficult to cite examples in the normal process of listening where *loudness* comparisons take a form similar to the task set for the listener in these intensity discrimination experiments. Perhaps in the field of music there is the greatest demand for the development of skill in producing controlled gradations in perceived loudness. Here we have a loudness scale, with at least the gross divisions identified, running from pianissimo (ppp) to fortissimo (fff) with possibly six labeled points between. There are also finer distinctions in subtle rhythmic and accent patterns. Whether these should be considered loudness judgments is subject to the same reservations just voiced. Perhaps these are rhythm and accent judgments and do not translate to loudness difference judgments simply because intensity change is one component involved.

Winckel (1967) reports an experiment that casts doubt on the agreement between musical loudness perception and loudness computed by the standard methods described. He had highly trained musicians, of the Cleveland Symphony, play a diatonic and a chromatic scale on their instruments keeping the loudness constant. The computed loudness of the resulting notes is far from constant.

All in all, loudness, taken into the laboratory, has not behaved as predictably as the basic nature of the intensity dimension would lead us to expect. One other factor that may have an effect is the necessity to process signals accurately in everyday listening in spite of the fact that their loudness varies widely from time to time and from one listening environment to another. Perhaps we learn not to be too dependent on preservation of precise differences in loudness.

9 Temporal Patterns

For the auditory analyzer operating as a sensory channel, the registering of time patterns in various meaningful signals is probably the most important task of all. Auditory signals that do not change with time are seldom useful to the organism, and we frequently adapt to them so completely as to be unaware that they continue. Furthermore, many sound sources of interest produce only very short sounds and their rate of change with time may be the most important parameter for their recognition.

This evidence of change in something in the environment is undoubtedly the most useful result of our analysis of sound. Also the sounds that we produce ourselves, such as speech and music, are characterized by continuous change, and the finer of these changes are more rapid than can be followed by our other sensory systems.

It is, in fact, surprising that the system can resolve as small intervals as it does. Though the speech articulators themselves move comparatively slowly, some of the discriminations of speech sounds made by the auditory analyzer depend on time differences of 10 msec or less. Similarly, the difference between good and excellent technique in performance on musical instruments may involve the same order of temporal discrimination. Perhaps location of sound sources by the binaural system epitomizes the limits of auditory time resolution. Here we need to deal in intervals of tens of microseconds to explain how we recognize that a sound source is displaced just a few degrees off center azimuth.

How can a neural network deal with such small intervals and the registering of such rapid patterns? We know there are some inherent limitations in temporal following. Lüscher and Zwislocki (1947) demonstrated long ago that when the ear is stimulated by even a very short tone, there is a subsequent interval during which the system does not respond as readily to a second stimulation. There is, in other words, a temporary shift of sensitivity, or threshold. Their method consisted of giving the ear a stimulating tone of 400 msec duration at a selected Sound Pressure Level and following this 20 msec later with a short test, or probe, tone. The frequency and time dimensions of this change in readiness to respond are shown in Fig. 36. This kind of temporal effect has since come to be known as forward masking—the interfering effect of a signal on a following signal; *i.e.*, the failure of the auditory system to separate two successive signals cleanly in time. Considering the pattern of excitation along the basilar membrane, both from physiological data and from other data on simultaneous interference or masking of tones, we might anticipate that a similar effect would also be seen for an immediately following tone of a closely adjacent frequency. That this is the case is apparent in Fig. 37 from Munson and Gardner (1950). Later work by Zwislocki and Pirodda (1952) verified this pattern and also indicated that at high intensities the maximum threshold shift is not at the frequency of the stimulating tone but as much as half an octave higher.

It is clear that the ability of the system to analyze rapidly changing time patterns, whether it be rapid repetitions at the same frequency or rapid successions of different frequencies, will be affected by the characteristics of forward masking—this failure of the system to recover immediately to its pre-signal state of readiness. The effects extend considerably beyond the 20 msec shifts shown in Fig. 36 A, but they do decay rapidly and are of greatest interest for the shortest post-stimulus intervals. The precise effects of tonal signals are very difficult to measure at these short intervals, since the shorter we make the tone the less restricted its frequency spectrum. Elliott (1962)

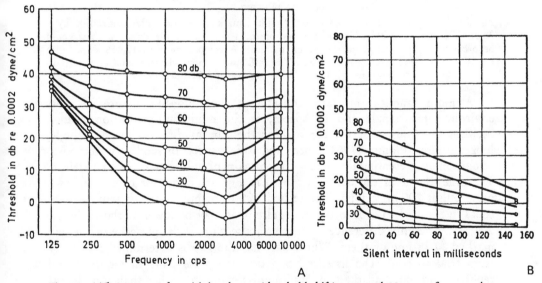

A   B

Fig. 36. *A* The amount of sensitivity change (threshold shift) measured 20 msec after cessation of a 400 msec tone. The numbers on the curve show the level of the stimulating tone. The amount of shift is measured by a very short burst at the same frequency. The bottom (unnumbered line) is the threshold for the short tone without any prior stimulation. *B* The change in threshold and the time course of return to normal threshold after stimulation of the ear with a 400 msec tone whose SPL is shown at the start of the curve. Even for fairly soft tones it takes ¹/₁₀ of a second before the ear has recovered its pre-tone sensitivity. Recovery is tested by giving a short test burst at the times shown on the abscissa. (From Lüscher und Zwislocki, 1947)

explored the forward masking of tones of three different frequencies by broad-band noise and showed that the change is indeed very rapid in this first 20 msec post-masker period. This change is portrayed later in Fig. 42.

The curves of Fig. 36 B were measured as the rate of return to normal sensitivity, but might also be viewed as the rate of decay of activity upon cessation of the previous stimulation. We have no way psychoacoustically of measuring the two aspects separately, or even of knowing if there are separate processes.

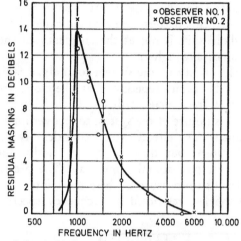

Fig. 37. The amount of threshold change (residual masking) 98 msec after stimulation by a 70 dB SPL tone at 1 kHz. The asymmetry of the pattern is in the direction that would be predicted by the peripheral excitation patterns. A comparison with Fig. 36 shows that partial recovery has already taken place. The shift just 10 msec after cessation of the 70 dB tone was nearly 35 dB. (From Munson and Gardner, 1950)

A more practical measure, considering the pulse-like nature of most environmental signals and of speech, is the minimum separation needed between two pulses for the ear to hear the pair as different from a single, longer pulse. Plomp (1964) measured this aspect of auditory temporal resolution by presenting listeners with two pairs of noise bursts for comparison. The time scheme of the bursts is shown in Fig. 38. Each pair consists of two noise pulses 200 msec long. The second 200-msec pulse of each pair may be equal in Sensation Level to the first pulse or it may be lower as shown in the diagram. The only difference in the two pulse pairs is the presence of the gap marked Δt in one of them. Which pair has the gap is determined randomly from trial to trial. The listener hears the two pulse pairs in sequence and reports which one had the gap. White noise was used rather than tone bursts because for such rapid changes it is not possible to say what place in the frequency range might give the clue to the presence of the gap.

As can be seen in Fig. 39, which shows the result for two listeners, the ability of the system to hear the second pulse depends on the strength of the first pulse, that is, on the remaining level of excitation. Presumably a second pulse of given strength is "hidden" in the decaying excitation from the first pulse until that excitation has decayed sufficiently.

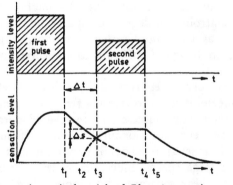

Fig. 38. The time pattern in a single trial of Plomp's experiment on decay rate. Δ t is varied to find the gap just noticeable to the listener. A separate set of trials is run for each level of the second noise pulse. At the bottom is a hypothetical scheme for the change in the level of auditory sensation during the noise-burst sequence. We know that it takes time for a burst of sound to reach its full loudness, so the sensation grows gradually. If decay time, Δ t, is very short, excitation is still high and a very weak pulse might not be heard. If the test pulse causes a change in excitation equal to the jnd in intensity, we might expect the test pulse to be detected. Thus the strength of the pulse needed at any time, t, after the end of the first noise pulse can lead to an estimate of how rapidly the excitation decays to threshold. (From Plomp, 1964b)

It is apparent from the graph that unless the first pulse is much stronger than the second, say more than 10 dB greater, gaps of the order of 3—5 msec are discernible by the auditory analyzer. It has also been shown with much shorter noise bursts (2 msec per burst) that a gap of 0.5 msec can be detected (Penner, 1977). This degree of resolution certainly goes beyond that needed to process the plosive and fricative sounds of speech.

It would be highly useful to have a similar estimate of auditory resolution for impulse sounds in the environment—the pops and clicks from which we

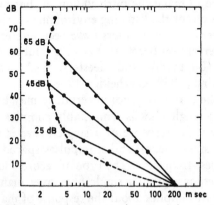

Fig. 39. The just noticeable silent gap between the two pulses in Fig. 38. The level of the first pulse is shown for each solid line. The level of the second pulse was varied as shown on the ordinate. As predicted, the longer the decay (silent) interval, the softer the just noticeable pulse. These lines must be closely related to the decay rate of auditory sensation. The dashed line shows the just noticeable silent gap for two bursts of equal sensation level. (From Plomp, 1964b)

learn what kinds of impacts are occurring. We might take two sharp clicks that can be finely controlled in degree of separation and see at what spacing the ear hears them as two clicks rather than one. This seemingly simple experiment proves to be quite difficult to interpret for reasons that are inherently very interesting.

Whenever the auditory system is presented with a closely-spaced repetition of a previous waveform, it tends to fuse the two into a single perception. This fusion is accomplished more successfully by the binaural system than the monaural, but it occurs even for monaural listening. If this were not the case we probably would hear separate echoes of impulse sounds even in small rooms rather than only in large spaces. Since the system performs this fusion of waveform copies, we hear separate echoes only when the spacing between original and repetition has reached about 30—50 msec (Haas, 1949; Lochner and Burger, 1958). With smaller spacings we do hear a difference between hearing the original alone and the original-plus-copy, but we ascribe the difference to the nature of the acoustic environment we're listening in. Sounds in a large room have a different quality because the walls are further away, the reflections take longer to get back to us, and the "copies" are more widely spaced. In a room with absorptive boundaries (draperies, carpets, etc.) the reflections are more attenuated than in a reverberant room, and again the sound of the room is different.

All this is a highly adaptive interpretation of time pattern analysis by the auditory system, but it certainly complicates the performing and the interpretation of the two-click experiment. We have already seen that presenting two equal-amplitude clicks gave rise to a pitch sensation when the click spacing was between 10 msec and 0.3 msec (McClellan and Small, 1967). Those listeners were not attending at the time to the single or double aspect of the click pair, but considering the versatility of the system they might be able to make both judgments. Many listeners, if the second click is actually the reflection from a wall, may not be able to make the pitch judgment, but instead relate the pair spacing to the dimensions of the listening environment—the acoustic coloration of the room. A number of experimenters *have* been interested in the separation point at which the perception becomes that of a double image, but the results are not unequivocal (Buytendijk and Meesters, 1942; Wallach, Newman and Rosenzweig, 1949; Hirsh, 1959; Gescheider, 1966).

Perhaps part of the reason for such uncertainty may be that the activity in the cochlea for even a single click is remarkably complex. When a click is fed to the ear of a cat and the response of a single nerve is recorded, the record shows, rather than a single neural spike, impulses spaced at the characteristic period of the fiber's best frequency. The type of record shown in Fig. 40 comes from accumulating response from a single fiber over many clicks, but we can picture roughly what this implies about the response of many similar fibers to a single click. One thing that must be added to the complexity is the fact that in response to a sharp click, which contains energy at many frequencies, different parts of the basilar membrane move at different times, according to the time pattern of the traveling wave.

In spite of this multiple activity, a single sharp click delivered to the

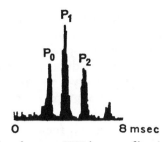

Fig. 40. Histogram of impulses from an VIIIth nerve fiber in response to a repeated click. Zero marks the time that each click was delivered at the input. The fiber does not always respond at the same delay time after the click but at several times which are spaced by the period $\left(\dfrac{1}{\text{characteristic frequency}}\right)$ of the fiber. (From Kiang, 1965)

auditory system still sounds punctate in time, and fine differences in click pairs can be discriminated. Since presumably any differences, that can be reliably heard may be useful to the system we need not restrict our inquiry about minimum discriminable difference between click pairs to the hearing of a double *vs* single image, but search instead for the smallest separation for which a *difference* can be reported. Something happens at about a 2 msec spacing which subjects tend to call roughness. Sometimes this has been taken to indicate separation, but if one actually asks the subject to designate when the image has become double the reports range all the way from 6 or 7 msec to about 50 msec. In view of the much finer time intervals the system *can* discriminate, it looks as though an active fusion of the two clicks by the system is taking place even for monaural listening.

Our question about minimum discriminable time interval, then, should take the form of ascertaining the smallest temporal change for which *some* difference can be heard. Since changing the spacing between pairs also changes the duration of the pair, we need a technique that will eliminate that possible clue. Ronken (1970) devised such a technique by presenting two clicks of unequal amplitude and presenting them in both orders before asking for a judgment. His listeners got the sequence shown in Fig. 41 and were asked to tell whether pair 1 and pair 2 sounded the same or different. The spacing between members of the pair was changed from trial to trial and the order was changed randomly. The great usefulness of this pattern is that nothing differs

Fig. 41. The signal sequence used by Ronken to measure minimum time resolution for clicks. On each listening trial two such click-like signals were presented. The listener responded only Same or Different. On half the trials the same signal is presented twice. On the other half (randomly determined) the second signal is the reverse of the first. The spacing between the strong and the weak peak is varied from trial to trial. When the time between peaks is so small that the listener can tell the difference only 75 % of the time, we have reached a limit of time resolution for peak spacing. If the amplitude ratio between peaks is changed, the results will differ somewhat

between the two pairs presented on a trial except the time pattern of the waveform. The energy spectrum of each pair and the duration are precisely the same. Ronken reported that when the spacing between individual clicks was 2 msec observers could hear correctly a difference between the two pairs 75 % of the time. Performance is not strongly dependent on relative height of the two members of the pair; if one pulse is somewhere around half the height of the other the discrimination can be successfully made. Later Resnick and Feth (1975) employed the same technique and found that for their optimum level (45 dB SL) and click-height ratio (1.4 : 1) the pair reversal could be discriminated at click spacings of 0.5 msec.

This is a most impressive degree of temporal resolution for the auditory system. But Hall and Lummis (1973) carried the same technique one step further. They used a masking noise with a gap centered at 2 kHz. Presumably only the unmasked segment of the basilar membrane contributed to the perceived click response. With a click-pair spacing of 250 μsec, which is half the period of the characteristic frequency at the location of the noise gap, detection threshold was different for the strong-weak pair than for the weak-strong pair.

What makes this degree of temporal resolution even more puzzling is a demonstration by Duifhuis (1973) that for short signals some sort of apparently-transient-related activity persists for as much as 75 msec after the signal itself. We know, of course, that some part of the system is in a different state than before the signal or no comparison with a second signal would be possible. The question is whether that part of the system that should be ready to respond to a different signal still shows some change after this long interval since resolution can be shown for such a short interval. Is there provision for something like time multiplexing in the system that we do not yet see with our rather gross methods of exploration?

Whether the same fine time sequence is useful to the auditory system in practical listening is a moot point without further work. From the observation of the finest discriminations we make in analytical listening, the demands we make on our high-fidelity transducers and the ability to distinguish musical instruments that otherwise appear identical, such excellent temporal performance seems reasonable.

But the evidence for such a high degree of temporal resolution is made even more puzzling by the fact that some interference takes place in the unexpected direction also. There is evidence of backward masking—the inability to detect the presence of a signal that comes *before* the masker and would be heard without the masker present. Miller (1947) first showed this for short tone bursts, but it has since been demonstrated for tone bursts in noise, clicks, and noise in noise, among others. For the masking of probe tones that precede the onset of a broadband noise, backward masking has the time form shown in Fig. 42 (Elliott, 1971). One explanation for this seemingly anomalous phenomenon is that stronger signals, which have been often demonstrated to have shorter latencies very early in the system, reach the processor as soon as some weaker preceding signals. A more teleologically oriented explanation is that weak signals are purposely suppressed when contiguous with strong ones.

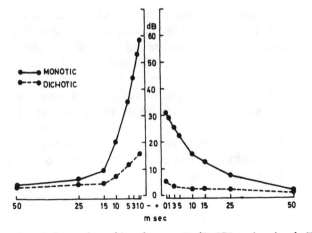

Fig. 42. Backward and forward masking from a 90 dB SPL noise signal. The noise was 50 msec in duration and the test probe to measure remaining threshold shift was a 5 msec 1 kHz tone pip. Left of the center line is shown the change in threshold for the tone pip at the times shown *preceding* the onset of the noise signal. To the right of the center line are results from measuring sensation level of the probe for the times after the end of the noise signal. The dashed line shows the results when the noise signal is in one ear and the test probe in the other. When weaker noise signals are used, the pattern is the same, but the amount of threshold shift is less. (From Elliott, 1962)

In our present state of ignorance, both these possibilities must be entertained.

But even though both forward and backward masking seem to smear the time domain to some extent, the auditory system does well in recognizing differences in even fairly rapid time patterns. We have looked at the evidence from two clicks. A number of measures of other signals indicate essentially the same thing. For very short tone bursts, where one tone starts 2 to 3 msec before the other the system can hear a difference when the starting order is changed (Patterson and Green, 1970; Efron, 1973). For a pattern of three consecutive short tones, Divenyi and Hirsh (1974) trained their listeners to tell which of the six possible 3-note permutations had been presented, even when the tones were as short as 2 msec. Performance was best when the 3-note "melody" covered a range greater than $1/3$ octave (musical major third—just about the width of the critical band) and when the three frequencies were harmonically related.

Much of the study of the limits of temporal resolution has taken the form of exploring forward and backward masking separately. Zwicker (1976) uses a dynamic masking paradigm that includes both. The masker in his experiments was a low frequency tone, and the probe tone was a short high frequency burst inserted in selected phases of the masker. The question is whether different amounts of masking of the probe tone will occur at different phases of the probe tone, for instance at positive peak, zero crossing or negative peak. Amount of masking does indeed follow the form of the low frequency wave, being greatest around the rarefaction maxima and least around the condensation maxima. This in itself furnishes interesting information about masking, but our immediate interest is in whether this following of the waveform coincides with our other estimates of temporal resolution. Zwicker reported that peaks and valleys in the masking pattern coinciding with the variation of the sinusoidal waveform of the masker did not fade out completely until the frequency of the masker was between 500 and 1000 Hz, *i.e.*, until the spacing between peaks and valleys was between 1 msec and 0.5 msec. This agrees surprisingly well with other estimates of auditory temporal resolution. It stops at about the same point as the following of rate change in interrupted white noise (see Pitch discussion) which has been for a long time taken as psycho-acoustic evidence for the limit of time-pattern following. It should be noted also that Zwicker's masking results indicate interaction of tones separated by much more than the critical band.

Fusion of Signals

Since the auditory system can discriminate such fine differences in temporal interval perhaps it also registers longer temporal patterns for further processing. Let us return to the problem of the failure to hear echoes even when the copy of the original is spaced by 10 msec or more after the original. This is ample separation for resolution into two separate patterns by the auditory system, and it would be difficult for us to contend, in the light of these results on discrimination of closely-spaced pulses, that the echo is being *masked* by the original. The experiment to test to what degree this happens with monaural addition of original waveform and copy has not been done, to my knowledge, but the conclusion is implied from binaural fusion of the two: the system must register and store the time pattern in sufficient detail and over a long enough period to fuse the two (or more) copies rather than separate them.

Most of the measurements on perception of the echo effect have been made on the speech signal. Auditory processing of speech is so complex that it is difficult to analyze the process. The same, or a comparable, fusing of echoes apparently takes place for other signals, since they too take on perceptually the coloration attributable to the acoustic properties of a room. Some help in interpretation comes from an experiment with random noise done with earphones, and relevant to the question of storage of the temporal pattern of a waveform (Blodgett *et al.*, 1956). A little preliminary explanation is in order: If we put the same random waveform into both earphones, what most observers report is a noise that seems to be in the center of the head. On the other hand, if we take noise from two separate noise generators and feed one to each ear, keeping the average level about the same, the noise will seem to be out at the two headphones. If feed the noise from the generator to, say, the right ear and then introduce a waveform delay of about a millisecond when putting that same noise in the left ear, all the sound seems to be at the right (leading) ear. Suppose we stretch the delay out to 5 milliseconds. Subjectively, the noise is still at the leading ear. Internally, the system recognizes that the lagging ear is a copy of the first waveform, but it does not report an echo;

instead it apparently fuses the two waveforms. It must have a running sample of the constantly changing time pattern going to each ear. How far can we offset the waveform pattern in the two ears and still get a single, fused impression at the leading ear? The listeners of the Blodgett et al. experiment showed considerable variability, but the good performers could still fuse the two copies at delays of 20 msec. The experimenters also report that the listeners who fused the longer delays were best at binaural localization judgments that require processing of extremely *small* interaural time differences. Cherry and Taylor (1954) reported that when one performs the same sequence with speech signals at the two ears, the outcome is very nearly the same. A single speech image appears at the leading ear until the lagging ear is about 20 msec behind, and at that point the image tends to separate into two. Whatever the system does to fuse the two copies seems to be independent of familiarity with the signal. Storage of some transformation of the waveform time pattern does appear to be the answer.

Is 20 msec the maximum length of some temporary waveform storage in the auditory processor? Hirsh's study (1959) of the perceived temporal order of two different auditory events indicated about 20 msec difference in onset was required before order could be reliably reported. We now know there are many exceptions to this, but it is interesting that for long signals and unfamiliar comparisons the fusion interval and the order-perception interval appear to be the same.

But we know from the work of Guttman and Julesz (1963) that 20 msec is not the longest random waveform sequence that can be recognized as a repetition. They repeated random sequences in a continuous chain, each link being a repetition of the same random noise sample, and listened for different impressions as the links in the chain were made longer. The most convincing type of signal for this purpose is a two-state waveform with equal probability of either state at any instance. This means that, at least in the input signal, the amplitude envelope or strong single peaks are not a clue. When such sequences were no longer than 50 msec and were repeated end to end the sound had a pitch. This agrees, as we have seen, with some other estimates of the lower limit of pitch. Longer than 50 msec, out to a single-repeated-segment length of 250 msec, a sound like the slow putt-putting of a motor was suggested, and for longer sounds something like whoosh-whoosh describes the sequence. With enough concentration by the listener, such random sequences can be recognized as repetitive out to a segment length of 2 sec. If we look on this as some form of auditory memory for time pattern it must be noted that it is a very restricted investigation of time-pattern storage. Guttman and Julesz made no effort to see how few repetitions were required to recognize the repetitive nature of the signal.

Why this task of picking up repetition of random patterns with durations of a second or so requires such concentration is a matter of some interest. Seemingly similar repetitions of unfamiliar waveforms do not present that difficulty. One can imagine, for example, water dropping on a resonant object not familiar to the listener. The system has no difficulty recognizing the similarity of the repetition even with a spacing of several seconds and would quickly note any change in the sound. Yet consecutive noise bursts lasting, say, 100 msec with a silent gap between could have a completely different waveform on each repetition and all sound alike. Pfafflin and Mathews (1966) tried training their subjects to recognize 12 different 96 msec noise bursts much as one would learn any other set of sounds. After over 100 trials on each noise, subjects were scoring about 50 % correct, getting some noises always correct and performing at chance on others. Just as we might predict for a good sensory system, the memorizing of time patterns that have no other associations, no intrinsic value, is not an easy task.

Spectrum Analysis 10

The ability of the auditory system to assign a pitch to signals that occupy either a point or a restricted segment of the spectrum is one important aspect of frequency analysis. Two other aspects of spectral shape must concern us in our effort to describe the manner in which the system differentiates and recognizes the various sounds useful to the organism. The first of these is the necessity to generate a different perception whenever the *pattern* of spectral distribution of energy changes to some differentiable degree. The second is some understanding of how the system succeds in recognizing two (or more) such spectral shapes when they are present simultaneously.

Sound Quality

Simply described, the first operation has to do with the relation between spectrum and the perception of sound quality, or timbre. We must note immediately that to tie quality or timbre exclusively to spectral pattern will lead to some difficulty. Evidence is already growing that rate of change of these patterns with time has a pervading effect on what we have traditionally included under the perception of sound quality. But for convenience, we will look first at effects that are present for unchanging steady-state complex sounds.

Initially, for further simplification, we may suppose that many sound sources of interest can be described as a generator of a complex waveform coupled to one or more resonators. This is not as restrictive as it may first sound because, as we may remember from some elementary physics, almost any mechanical device with both mass and stiffness will have a resonant frequency.

$$f_r = \frac{1}{2\pi} (S/M)^{1/2}$$

It follows from the formula that if the more dominant of these two properties of an object is its mass it will resonate to a low frequency, other things being equal; and if the device is primarily stiff and not very massive its resonant frequency will be high. What must be included for our purposes is the fact that this applies also to air columns and other enclosed or partially enclosed volumes of air. When their stiffness in displacement per unit of force and their mass are both expressed in the proper units, their resonant frequency is predicted from the same expression. How sharp the resonance, or the tuning, will be depends on the relative amount of frictional or viscous resistance in the device, but even if the device is heavily damped with resistance, its resonant frequency is still predicted approximately from the above expression. We can see that most devices when set into either transient or steady vibration might be said to have one or more characteristic frequencies. The characteristic frequency of an VIIIth nerve fiber, of course, has nothing to do with these properties of the nerve, but only with the mechanical properties of the segment of membrane where it originates.

Before looking further at the auditory effects of the behavior of these resonances, we should note that differences in the waveform that drives the resonator(s) may also have some predictable influence on the resulting spectrum, and therefore on the auditory response. If, for example, the driving waveform is a series of sharp pulses as in (C) of Fig. 43 the partials, or harmonics, are of nearly equal strength, as shown. If it is a square wave, as in (B) it contains only the odd harmonics, dying away in amplitude with increasing harmonic number as shown.

Now, these waveforms, as the period (time taken for a single repetition) is lengthened or shortened, keep the same relative strength for each of the harmonics. This constancy of spectral nature of the source will contribute a certain characteristic quality. Most laboratory workers are familiar with the reedy, hollow sound of the square wave, or the "buzzy" character of the train of sharp pulses.

How strong a contribution this constancy of relations among the partials makes to the judgment of the quality of a complex sound is difficult to say. We looked for a partial answer in our own laboratory by choosing some complex waveforms that would not be expected to be familiar to listeners, since they were simply random tracings repeated so many times per second. Since they are different waveforms they have a different spectrum, *i.e.*, a different pattern of relative strengths of the harmonics, and therefore a different sound quality. But suppose we move this pattern up the spectrum by changing the repetition rate—increasing the fundamental frequency. Does the sound quality really remain unmistakably the same? The question can be answered experimentally by giving the listener a pair of sounds with the fundamental frequency always changed for the second member of the pair. Sometimes the waveform will also be changed for this member, sometimes waveform will remain the same and only the fundamental frequency will change. If the subjective quality remains strongly the same in spite of changing fundamental frequency, listeners will always be able to tell which pairs had waveform *and* frequency changed for the second member and which

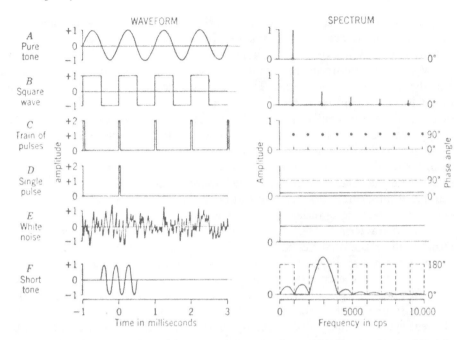

Fig. 43. A short review of waveform and spectrum. The amplitude spectrum is shown by vertical lines, the phase spectrum by dots or dashed lines. The sine wave *(A)* has a spectrum portrayed as energy at a single frequency. By convention a sine wave that has a positive-going zero crossing at time zero is in sine phase (see dot on base line). A square wave spectrum *(B)* consists of only odd harmonic partials. If we call the amplitude of the fundamental 1, then the amplitude of the nth partial is 1/n. To make a square wave these are added in sine phase. A repeated train of pulses *(C)*—in this case one per millisecond—has harmonic partials spaced 1 kHz apart. Viewing this as a sum of sinusoidal components makes it apparent that all sinusoids must peak at time zero, therefore they are all in cosine phase. If the pulse is sharp enough all harmonic partials will have nearly the same amplitude as shown. A single pulse *(D)* will have energy spread continuously through the spectrum. If we view it as the sum of infinitely closely spaced sinusoids they would all have cosine phase. White noise *(E)* is a randomly varying waveform, and its long-term spectrum is also continuously and evenly distributed over the spectrum with phase random. The spectrum of a short tone burst *(F)* is important in audition. Its phase spectrum is seldom of interest, but it changes polarity as shown every 1/T Hertz where T is the duration of the burst. (From Licklider, 1951)

ones had only the frequency changed. The question is whether they can recognize constancy of waveform in spite of a change in fundamental frequency. The outcome was that if the fundamental was changed only a little, listeners could tell whether the waveform was the same or changed. But if the fundamental changed by as much as a musical tone, listeners could tell only 75 % of the time whether the quality, as defined by waveform, had stayed the same.

What, then, does make the perceived quality of a sound source remain the same as the fundamental frequency changes? The best examples come from musical instruments. As suggested earlier, they are characterized by one or more resonance regions. In general, this will mean that the spectral region of the resonance will continue to be emphasized in spite of changes in the fundamental. In both musical instruments and in the voice these characteristic resonance regions are called formants. Their presence probably contributes heavily to the quality of most familiar sound sources.

With many environmental sources of sound the situation is less simple, but the same principle holds. The characteristic resonant behavior of an object is what identifies it for the auditory system. Frequently, however, the object will be subjected to an impulsive blow rather than being driven by a steady waveform. Out of the great variety of such sounds, we select some invariant audible characteristic(s). We recognize when the sound has come from the striking of a can, a bottle or a table in spite of considerable variation in size and material. For poorly tuned sources, the time sequence of events gets more important. We recognize aurally the size and structure of closing doors or of breaking branches, for instance.

Thus characteristic frequency identification is an important part of the recognition of the qualities that identify what it is that made a sound. It is in one sense a step beyond the recognition of pitch alone that we inspected in chapter 7. In the case of driven sources, such as musical instruments, we recognize both the pitch being produced (usually fundamental frequency) and the quality or timbre of the sound. Most frequently this latter takes the form of identifying (naming) the source by its spectral pattern; it is a clarinet, or like a clarinet, etc. But we also have some more abstract terms to characterize the quality of sounds. They may be dull, hollow, mellow, strident, etc. But how do these terms relate to the components in, or the shape of, the spectrum? One of the most comprehensive attempts to systematize these responses is a study by von Bismarck (1974). He took 30 descriptive pairs of adjectives and applied them to 35 different shapes of steady-state spectrum. These are schematized in Fig. 44. Judgments were elicited for each adjective pair on each tone by eight musically trained and eight musically untrained subjects in a 7-point semantic differential pattern.

Factor analysis methods were used to identify four factors that appear to account for a large proportion of the listener's responses. The two of these that account for a large proportion of the variance von Bismarck called "sharpness" and "compactness". This seems an imaginative approach to the problem of unifying the description of sound quality, but to see the basic difficulty one needs to ask how often we hear sounds discussed in terms of their sharpness or compactness.

Some further thought convinces us that what we do much more frequently when asked to describe an unfamiliar sound is to liken the sound in question to some other—possibly more familiar, sound source. And, indeed, this is what we might expect from a sensory system whose primary assignment is to inform the organism what is happening to sound sources of interest. It is much more important for this system to recognize common elements and assign similar sources to the same class than to apply labels which may have little to do with the actual function of the sound source.

Von Bismarck's complex tones had none of the characteristic attack and decay properties of everyday sources of sound. Very likely for a set which *did* include these additional clues, the tendency to ascribe the sound to familiar

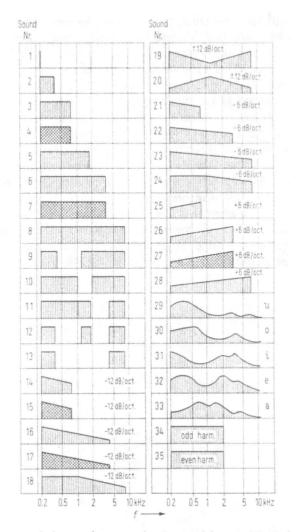

Fig. 44. The 35 spectral shapes of tones and noises used by von Bismarck to analyze the perceptual factors in sound quality. Vertical striations indicate tonal (line spectrum) signal at a 200 Hz fundamental. Stippled areas indicate noise signals.
(From von Bismarck, 1974)

vibrating objects with similar sound-producing properties would be even stronger.

Grey (1977) accomplished a formal multivariate analysis of the perceptual similarities of musical tones including normal attack and decay characteristics. Temporal characteristics, particularly attack characteristics and synchronicity of partials, played a heavy role in the assignment of musical tones to perceptually similar classes or families of sounds or sound sources. Basically, the auditory system performs best as an identifier of sound sources and what those sound sources are doing or having done to them. (Schubert, 1975; Huggins, 1953.)

But even without time clues, and without the requirement of identifying the tone, it takes very little change in a steady-state complex tone for the system to hear a small difference in quality, or timbre. The Seashore Test of Musical Aptitude included a test of the smallest change in relative strengths of the partials of a complex tone. A change of 1 dB in only one of eight harmonic partials can be detected as a slight change in timbre by the most sensitive ears.

Thus far we have spoken only of the relative amplitudes of the different harmonic partials of a complex tone. One question that arises is whether the auditory system responds directly to that aspect of the spectrum or whether relative phase of the partials also makes a difference in the perception of a sound. A fundamental tenet in the synthesis of complex sounds is that any periodic sound is the sum of integer-related sinusoids. This is simply illustrated in Fig. 45. But it is apparent that if we shifted the phase of one or more of the sinusoids by other than a full period (of that partial) the complex waveform would no longer be the same. So far as overall waveform is concerned the change might be as drastic as the contrast in Fig. 46, which shows one wave-

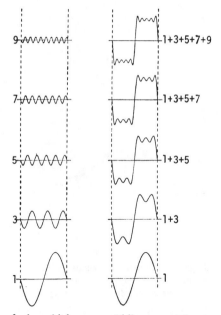

Fig. 45. An example of sinusoidal waves adding to make a complex periodic wave. In this case an approximate square wave can be synthesized from just harmonic partials 1, 3, 5, 7 and 9. Adding still more odd-numbered partials with the right amplitude and phase relation would bring the resultant even closer to a square wave. (See Fig. 43)

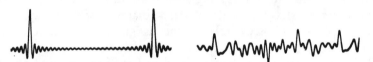

Fig. 46. The waveform on the left results when 15 harmonic partials are added in cosine phase (see Fig. 43). The waveform on the right is the sum of the same sinusoids but with phase relations among them completely random

form resulting from all tones in cosine phase (all reaching a maximum at instant t_0) and another from tones of the same relative amplitude but with randomly selected phase relations. With this great a difference in phase (waveform?) the two complex sounds have a different quality, the cosine waveform having more of a buzzer-like quality. Their pitch does not change.

Does a difference in the phase relation of the partials always make a difference in auditory perception? Quite a number of studies have simplified the question by presenting only two partials, usually 1st and 2nd, and asking whether changes in their relative phase can be heard. In general, the answer is that changing phase in such steady-state tones makes a scarcely perceptible difference auditorally. But we must remember that for short tones or for rapidly-changing tones phase, time and frequency are not so easily separated, and there we need to re-assess whether the phase characteristics of sound sources and sound transmitting devices, including the ear itself, must be taken into account.

If the ear does recognize sounds and sound sources by analyzing a waveform into its spectral components and identifying the resultant pattern as energy distribution across the frequency range, then it does a remarkable job. One can hear the noise of a typewriter in the same room at the same time that the system picks up the sound of heels on the hard floor and simultaneously listens to the speech of someone talking in the vicinity. All these sounds are heard as though they arrive independently at the ears, and at least for uncritical listening, they appear essentially undistorted. They do not by any means occupy completely separate parts of the spectrum, yet only when the undesired one gets much stronger than the preferred one do they seem to interfere.

Listening to music furnishes even more impressive examples of the amazing ability to separate sounds which occupy partly overlapping portions of the spectrum. Most musical listeners can readily hear several instruments in an ensemble and can tell also if the quality of one or more of them is not conforming to an acceptable standard. Two familiar voices singing in unison can still be separated into the two recognizable qualities of each individual voice in many instances. As a dynamic, real-time spectrum analyzer, the system has no equal.

Simultaneous Masking

Even though these examples represent an impressive degree of spectral resolution, the system is by no means a perfect spectrum analyzer; and it is the degree of its failure to separate simultaneously present signals completely that tells much of what we do know about the nature of spectral analysis. Thus much of the study of this aspect of auditory behavior is occupied with the degree to which the reception of one signal changes in the presence of another—the masking of one signal by another.

In its simplest, most quantifiable form masking is defined as the change in detectability of one tone in the presence of another of specified level. We begin with tones because they occupy a single point on the frequency range, and we need specify only frequency and amplitude to describe the tone completely for our purposes.

The results of the early work of Wegel and Lane (1924) on the effect of one tone on tones of other frequencies is shown in Fig. 47. The method employed was to use one pure tone—in this case one at 1200 Hz—as the masker. This tone is present continually and the experiment consists of finding how much the level for minimum audibility (the threshold) of other tones has changed in the presence of this masker. We can get a general picture of how

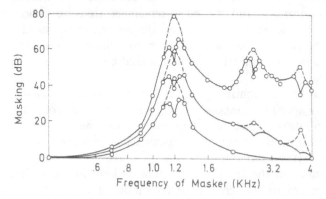

Fig. 47. The effect of a 1200 Hz tone on the audibility of other tones. The lowest curve indicates how much the presence of a 40 dB SL tone shifts the threshold for other frequencies. Below the curve only the 1200 Hz tone is audible. The middle curve is for a 60 dB tone, and the top curve for 80 dB Sensation Level. The uncertainty at 1200 Hz, 2400 Hz and 3600 Hz, indicated by the dashed curve, is attributable to the hearing of a beat-like phenomenon in these areas. (Modified from Wegel and Lane, 1924)

tones of other frequencies are affected, but even when the masker tone is at a comparatively low level some difficulty of interpretation arises at frequencies close to the masker. What happens when the two tones are too close, as we recall from an earlier discussion, is that the masker beats with the test tone, and thus the criterion for hearing the test tone is changed completely in that region. At high levels of the masker (see the curve marked 80 dB SL) difficulty arises also at integer multiples of the fundamental. Arguments have ensued about *why* beat-like phenomena occur at these points, but for our present purposes the salient point is that they interfere with our estimate of the masking pattern of a pure tone.

Egan and Hake (1950) reasoned that this beating effect might be considerably ameliorated if the masker used were a band of noise rather than another pure tone. Their band of noise was about 90 Hz wide. The masking curve, shown in Fig. 48, does avoid much of the problem, as is seen by contrasting it with the pattern for a tone at the same frequency as the peak of the noise. The masking area is still markedly asymmetrical, showing much more interference with tones above the masker than below. This is borne out by the general observation, made even by Mayer back in 1876, that low frequency sounds tend to interfere with high frequency sound, but the reverse is not found.

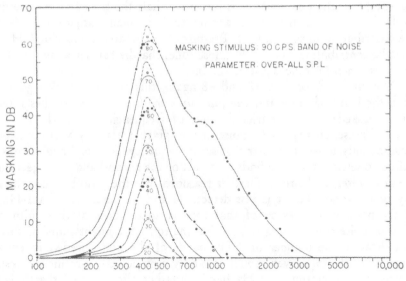

MASKING IN DB

FREQUENCY IN C.P.S.

MASKING STIMULUS: 90 C.P.S. BAND OF NOISE

PARAMETER: OVER-ALL S.P.L.

Fig. 48. Masking patterns of a narrow band of noise centered at 410 Hz. When the tone is near the center of the band a roughness clue gives an extra indication of the tone's presence. For this reason the dashed lines have been added. At extremely low levels, the patterns look nearly symmetrical. As the level rises the pattern seems more closely related to the neural patterns seen previously. It is as though the ≈ 400 Hz noise usurps fibers with higher characteristic frequencies and keeps frequencies above 400 Hz from being heard. (From Egan and Hake, 1950)

If we look back at the response areas of the individual fibers of the auditory nerve (see Figs. 16 and 23) we see that a fiber with a characteristic frequency f_c is much more likely to respond to frequencies lower than f_c than it is to frequencies above f_c. Therefore a strong low-frequency signal is likely to usurp (lock to its own frequency pattern, perhaps) fibers that have characteristic frequencies higher than its own frequency. We apparently have a neural basis for the shape of the masking pattern when the masker is a tone or a narrow band of noise.

Auditory Filters–Critical Bandwidths

How nearly is this masking behavior the same across the audible frequency range? Fletcher (1940) shaped a broad-band random noise shown in Fig. 49 so that it raised the threshold of any tone in the audible range by 50 dB. But note that the tones are not the same distance above the top of the noise. Each point on the curve of the noise portrays the Sound Pressure Level of the noise in a 1-Hz band at that frequency. This is defined as the Pressure Spectrum Level (L_{ps}) for a continuous-spectrum sound. We suspect, from the data of Fig. 47 and 48 that it is primarily the noise in the frequency range close to the tone that contributes to masking the tone. Perhaps the difference between the energy of the tone when it is just heard half the time and the energy in a 1-Hz band of the masker is a clue to how many adjacent 1-Hz bands are contributing to the masking. Presumably, a greater number of 1-Hz bands must be contributing to masking those tones that lie further above the level of the noise when the tone is just detectable.

Now if we check Figs. 47 and 48 again, this approach makes good sense. Both the band of noise and the pure-tone masker in these studies interfered with (masked) only a restricted range of frequencies. Similarly for a wide band of noise, energy in the noise at any given frequency will contribute to masking only tones at or near that same frequency. It is as though one is using a filter to select a tone and finds that part of the broad-band noise gets through the same filter as the tone. Fletcher reasoned that the ratio between the intensity of the tone when it is just detectable and the intensity of a 1-Hz band of the noise in the region of that tone is an estimate of the width of the band of noise contributing to masking the tone. We might think of this ratio as indicating the number of 1-Hz bands of the noise needed to equal the intensity of the tone, even though it is only a numerical convenience to specify a continuous spectrum in 1-Hz bands. Fletcher also assumed that it is when these two intensities are equal that the tone is just detectable in the noise.

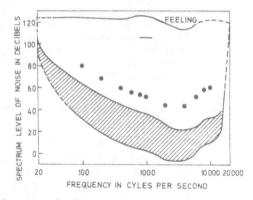

Fig. 49. The sound pressure level per cycle (spectrum level) of a noise that raises the threshold of all frequencies by 50 dB is shown by the line at the top of the shaded area. The lower curve is the sensitivity limit of the ear. The dots show the SPL of the tones when they are just audible in the presence of the noise. (From Fletcher, 1940)

In Fig. 49 we have the decibel difference between the tone when just masked and the pressure spectrum level at that same frequency. If we divide this decibel figure by 10 we have the logarithm of the number of 1-Hz bands required to make the intensity of the interfering noise equal the intensity of the tone. If Fletcher's assumption were correct—that the tone is just detectable when the energy of the tone and the energy of that part of the noise interfering with it are equal—then we would have an estimate of the width of the filter that is separating the rest of the noise from the tone. Subsequent work makes it appear that assumption is not tenable, so Fletcher's results are best designated as just what was measured—the ratio between the intensity of the tone and the intensity of a 1-Hz band of the masking noise, sometimes called the critical ratio. From Fig. 49, and from many subsequent measurements, it varies in width over the frequency range.

Is this width of the filter-like mechanism used to detect a tone in a broad noise a good estimate of the spectral resolution of the ear? Some time after the Fletcher report, Zwicker, Flottorp and Stevens (1957) described a set of experiments that cover a greater scope of spectral analysis and that do not depend on Fletcher's assumption of equal energy for tone and interfering noise. Those experiments and other work stemming from them have fixed rather firmly in audition the concept of a specific filter-like mechanism that apparently is early enough in the sequence of auditory analysis that it imposes the same bandwidth on many different operations. It is now common practice to speak of the critical-band filter, though we ought to remember that it is only a convenient analog or model for an auditory spectral analyzer that is much more versatile and adaptive than those we work with in the laboratory.

The work of Zwicker, *et al.* did establish some very convincing similarities between auditory analysis and laboratory filters. In one experiment they presented to the listener a closely spaced cluster of four tones, perhaps only 10 Hz apart. The listener matched the loudness of this narrow four-component signal to a single tone. If the spacing of the tones was made a little greater, the loudness match remained the same. But at a certain spacing, *i.e.*, beyond a certain width of the four-tone signal, it required a greater Sound Pressure Level of the single tone to maintain the loudness match. Why should this be? The energy of the four-tone complex has remained the same. A reasonable guess is that at the critical spacing there is less overall interference between the four tones, and it is convenient to say they are no longer completely encompassed in a single auditory filter. If we look at the spacing for which this loudness change occurs at different points over the frequency range, a plot of these spacings shows the same *shape* of curve as the Fletcher estimates for the critical ratio.

Masking behavior was also shown to follow the same form, through the following experiment (Zwicker et al., 1957). A narrow band of noise can be masked by a pair of tones on either side of the noise. This seems the reverse of the usual masking experiment. The narrow noise is turned on and off and the masking tones are constantly present. The listener indicates when he can hear the noise in the presence of the two tones. Having found the level at which the noise is just barely detectable, the experimenter can widen the spacing of the two tones and the noise signal will stay equally detectable—up to a point. That point, at which the noise now becomes more detectable, represents the same spacing as was found to yield the increase in loudness for the previous experiment. Again, the situation can be likened to placing a filter at the position of the wanted signal—in this case the noise band—and finding that when the interfering tones have moved outside the filter width the interference is less.

Since those experiments we have learned that quite a variety of auditory impressions change as we exceed the spacing of this critical bandwidth, among them the ability to hear two separate pitches when two sinusoids are present (Plomp, 1964; Haggard, 1970), the change from the impression of consonance to dissonance, the ability to hear the difference between amplitude modulation and frequency modulation, etc.

Similar measures for evidence of the operation of a critical band has come from a few experiments on animals (Watson, 1963; Pickles, 1975). The animals are trained to respond to tones that are minimally audible in the presence of noise; then the form of the experiment is parallel with the Fletcher derivation of critical ratios. This kind of critical-band function for the cat differs very little from that for the human. Thus far, however, attempts to relate the critical bandwidth to neurophysiological data have met with only limited success.

Since over much of the range the width is a constant ratio corresponding to about 1.2 : 1, other logarithmic variation shows an obvious parallel. Because frequency representation along the basilar membrane is approximately logarithmic, the constant frequency ratio of the critical band means each critical band spans a constant distance along the cochlea, namely about 1.2 mm. A frequency ratio of 1.2 is about a quarter of an octave ($2^{1/4} \approx 1.2$) and musically corresponds to an interval of a minor third.

In attempting as complete an understanding of the spectral resolution of the system as is possible, another technique has recently been explored—one that seems to outline the shape of the excitation pattern for a selected signal. As in masking measurements we begin with a strong low-frequency signal and a weak high-frequency signal, and the pattern of excitation might look like the diagram of Fig. 50. This might portray the situation in the cochlea

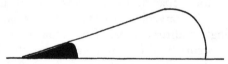

Fig. 50. Conceivable cochlear excitation pattern for a strong low-frequency signal and a weak high-frequency signal. The suggestion is that the high-frequency pattern is completely contained in the tail of the low-frequency distribution

or it could be further up the system. If the situation is as shown and two signals are alternated in time at appropriate rates, the amount of activity at the high frequency segment is the same for both signals. The reason for describing it in that fashion is that under the conditions outlined a particular ratio of strong to weak signal exists for which the weak signal *appears* continuous even though it is intermittent. This is designated as the pulsation threshold of the weak signal. It seems reasonable to believe this occurs because for the area excited by the weak signal excitation does not change appreciably for the two signals and it is therefore a measure of the excitation level attributable to the strong signal *at the location of the weak signal.* If we systematically present the same situation for signals of other frequencies in the presence of the same strong signal, we have one kind of estimate of the shape of the excitation pattern for the strong signal—another kind of masking pattern. This one is not subject to the problems of beating at frequencies close to the masker, and is not a detection threshold but a pulsation threshold.

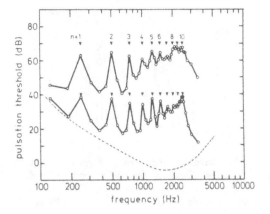

Fig. 51. The pulsation threshold for various test tones when alternated with a 250 Hz, ten partial complex tone. The partials are of equal amplitudes, as shown by the placement of the small triangles (70 dB SPL for one set of measurements, and 40 dB for the other). The minimum audibility curve for pure tones is shown as a dotted line.
(From Houtgast, 1974)

A convincing demonstration of the capabilities of the method comes from measuring the excitation pattern of a complex tone (Houtgast, 1974). The result is shown in Fig. 51. It agrees well with other estimates of the ear's ability to separate the lower partials of a complex tone. Relating this estimated shape of excitation pattern to estimates of critical bandwidth is not particularly easy.

Shape of Auditory Filter

Whatever the underlying mechanism may be, signals interact differently with each other when they are within a critical-band spacing than when they are outside it. This has a convenient descriptive similarity to a filter— our most common device for spectrum analysis. But if we find the filter analogy convenient we must recognize that specifying the filter width does not describe the filter sufficiently. To understand and predict its behavior for the various spectral analyses the ear performs, we ought to know the filter shape.

If we are assigned, in the laboratory, the task of finding the shape of a filter, the procedure is a standard one. Keeping the input amplitude to the filter constant as we vary the frequency, we plot the output amplitude as a function of frequency. But we know the auditory filter, whatever and wherever it may be, will literally not "sit still" for this operation. It insists on re-centering on such an input signal as the frequency is changed.

How, then, can we plot its shape? Patterson (1976) found a clever way to estimate the shape of the filter in spite of this problem. Suppose we hold the filter at a constant position by presenting the same tone rather than changing the input frequency. Then we gradually fill the filter with noise as suggested in the diagram of Fig. 52. When the noise has the large gap shown

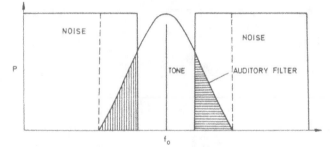

Fig. 52. Diagram of the increasing interference of noise with a tone centered in a filter. As the gap in the noise narrows from the dotted-line position to the solid-line position, more noise enters the filter and interferes with the tone. The level of the tone must be raised to remain audible (see text). (Modified from Patterson, 1976)

by the dashed lines, the threshold for the tone should be the same as without noise added. None of the noise is in the filter that is centered on the tone. If the noise is changed (the noise gap is narrowed) until its position is as shown by the solid lines, the threshold for the tone will rise because now some of the noise is in the same filter that is centered on the tone. How much the tone threshold changes is a measure of how much noise is inside that filter.

If we move the edge of the noise gap only slightly closer, we can, without too much error, regard the added noise-filled increment as a tall, narrow rectangle on each side underneath the filter. The successive heights of each of these rectangles as we gradually narrow the gap gives a piecewise approximation to the shape of the filter. Geometrically, the area of the rectangle is the frequency change (Δf) along the baseline times the average height of the filter curve at that point. But the area of each rectangle, *assuming filter symmetry*, is also equal to $1/2$ the added noise under the filter (ΔI) as given by the necessary increase in the tone to stay equally detectable. Thus for each change in the cutoff frequency of the noise, we have

$$h_i = \frac{\Delta I_{fi}}{2\Delta f}$$

where h_i is the height of the filter at a given point, and f_i is the center frequency of a given Δf

and the filter shape can be traced.

This derivation of the shape of the filter yields a curve something like the smoothed version shown in Fig. 52. In a later experiment, Patterson and Nimmo-Smith (1980) eliminated the bothersome symmetry assumption by measuring the amount of masking of the tone for different placements inside the noise gap and making the reasonable assumption that the system places the listening filter optimally for maximizing the signal to noise ratio. The equivalent rectangular width of the filters from Patterson's experiments agrees roughly with the widths from the Zwicker *et al.* set of measurements. There is no indication, however, of a marked inflection point around the width that emerges from so many quite difference auditory operations ($f_0 \pm 0.1$ on the graph).

From a comparison of physiological and psychoacoustic data, it seems reasonable to conclude that this degree of spectral analysis is accomplished at the level of the output of the cochlea (Evans and Wilson, 1973). Thus the critical bandwidth is a pervasive concept in assessing the ability of the ear to separate signals and in the masking of one signal by others. There is also ample evidence, both physiological and psychoacoustic, of direct inter-action of signals spaced wider than a critical band. Under these circumstances, even though spectral filtering of the order of the critical band takes place as early as the cochlea, parallel wide band processing should not be dismissed in an analyzer as complex as the auditory system.

11 Binaural Hearing

When we listen outside the laboratory, sounds definitely appear to be at the sound source. When a door closes, the sound is subjectively at the doorway, the typewriter noise is at the typewriter, etc. We may speak analytically of the sound reaching our ears, but only under unusual conditions do we actually get that subjective impression. This is a very fortunate state of affairs, for it greatly enhances the usefulness of the auditory sensory input. Let's inspect this aspect of hearing a little more broadly. When we listen in the usual environment, the location of several sound sources is usually automatically and simultaneously apparent. As I write this, the sounds of traffic through a window on my left seem quite distinct spatially from the constant whirring of a computer fan through the door in front of me, and I need make no effort to separate these from the sounds in a secretary's office through a door to my right. I have around me an auditory space nearly as useful to me as the more intuitively obvious visual space. The comparison is not really seriously intended; the two spaces are complementary, not competitive.

Much of the naturalness and the usefulness of this auditory space depends on the presence of two ears rather than one. Localization of sounds is possible with one ear, but both from subjective reports and from our analysis of the principles of sound localization we know that both accuracy and scope of spatial awareness suffer with only one ear operating.

Localization of Sound

Location of sound source with two ears seems fairly simple if we start with sources in a horizontal plane around the level of the ears. Starting with sinusoidal sounds we can note that changes in two simply-specified clues correspond to changes in location of the source in that plane. First of all, we can agree to ignore differences in distance for the moment by restricting our source locations to the circumference of a circle with the head at the center. We can also assume, in this first approach, that the head is a sphere and the existence of the pinna can be temporarily ignored. Finally, we will take no account, in this initial formulation, of reflection from the usual boundaries. This corresponds to the situation depicted in Fig. 53. If the source is close to the head the difference (D) in path length to the two ears is

$$D = r\,(2\theta)$$

where r is the radius of the sphere (head), and θ the departure from zero (front) azimuth. If the source is far enough from the head that the assumption of parallel paths to the sides of the head can be made, the difference is approximated by

$$D = r\,(\theta + \sin\theta).$$

Frequently the situation of interest will lie between these two, but for simplicity we will adopt the latter expression. Since distance divided by speed gives the travel time, dividing D by the speed of sound will give us the additional time for the longer path, or the delay time (τ) between ears. These values as azimuth of the sound source changes (zero azimuth being the direction the nose points) are plotted as the lower dashed line in Fig. 54. The higher dashed line is the predicted τ from the diffraction of a steady pressure difference around the head.

The solid lines represent data from a number of experiments with tones and clicks, measuring the delay on artificial or real heads with microphones at the position of the ears. Click data adhere quite closely to the geometric prediction; the tones show the effects of the increasing operation of diffraction as lower frequencies are measured.

From physical considerations alone we might expect that time difference between ears is a useful clue for pure tones only up to certain frequencies. We must note first of all that for any periodic signal if τ is the delay between

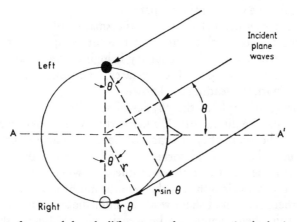

Fig. 53. Geometry for a path-length difference to the two ears in the horizontal plane. The line A—A′ is the line of 0° azimuth. In the situation shown, the left is the leading ear and the right the lagging ear

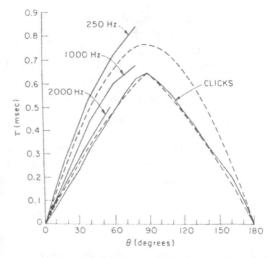

Fig. 54. Interaural delay times (τ) for tones and clicks. The data for tones, shown by the solid lines, are from interaural phase-difference measurements by a number of investigators. The click data hang close to the second formula in the text, which plots as the lower dashed line. The upper dashed line is D = r (3 sinΘ). (From Durlach and Colburn, 1978)

peaks in the leading and lagging ear, then period-minus-τ is the delay between the lagging ear and the peak of the next cycle. Since lead and lag ear are *our* designation, not known to the auditory system, either of these two values could be the delay between ears. Suppose we try a likely example: The period of 1 kHz (one millisecond) is already of the order of the maximum travel distance between ears. If we check the value of τ for an azimuth of 90° (sound source opposite one ear) the time between ears is about 600 μsec. If a peak of our 1 kHz sinusoid is arriving at left ear 600 microseconds later than at the right it is also just about 400 μsec earlier than the next peak at the left ear. Is the sound directly opposite the right ear (600 μsec later at the left); or is it 35° off center to the left (abscissa value for 400 μsec on 1 kHz curve)? Either of these fits the interaural time pattern.

The system can either (a) read only the smaller of the two intervals, or (b) supplement the time clue with other information about which ear is leading. In any event, when the frequency is high enough that the travel time between ears equals one period or greater, the time clue alone will be ambiguous even with the leading ear known.

An interesting principle of the physics of sound comes to our rescue as the efficacy of the time cue diminishes. We know that when sound waves encounter an obstacle like the head, they diffract, or bend, around the obstacle. This is what enables us to hear around corners as well as we do. But for an obstacle like a sphere (or the head), at those frequencies where the obstacle is large compared to the wavelength of the sound much more of the sound is reflected and there is a sound shadow at the immediate far side of the obstacle. The result of this phenomenon can be seen in Fig. 55. Sound shadow can be viewed as roughly analogous to the more familiar light shadow, namely less intensity per unit area in the shaded locations. From the figure we see some evidence of a sound shadow at 500 Hz, since, when the source is at the side rather than the front (azimuth=90°) level at the far ear is about 5 dB less than at the near ear. Note, however, that the slope of the 500 Hz line is nowhere very great, hence for small changes in location of the source (azimuth), the concomitant change in amplitude ratio at the two ears might not be discernible by the auditory system. At 5000 Hz, however, the situation has changed. The shadow cast is much sharper and the change per degree of azimuth is correspondingly increased. These curves are taken on human heads, and the shapes remind us these are not perfect spheres, nor are the pinnas symmetrical from front to back.

A more complete portrayal of the change in the maximum interaural sound ratio as frequency changes is seen in part b of the figure. From these measurements we would predict that at high frequencies the amplitude difference between ears might furnish a usable clue to the position of the sound source in the horizontal plane. We know that with earphones, where we can be reasonably certain that an intensity difference is the only interaural difference, a 3 dB difference will definitely move the perceptual image toward the ear with the stronger signal.

Incidentally, much of the interest in exploring localization of sound has centered on assessing the interaural time and intensity cues separately. In order to do so one must deliver the sound through earphones, and a dramatic perceptual change takes place. Whenever the ordinary binaural listening situation is altered, that is, when time, intensity and visual clues do not combine realistically, the sound image is perceived as either inside the head or on an arc just to the rear of the head. Manipulation of this sound image by control of time and intensity cues has been defined as the study of lateralization rather than localization. This is a useful distinction—one that should be carefully observed.

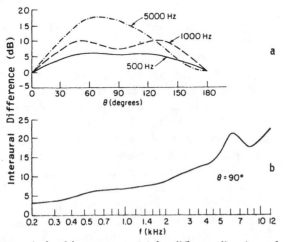

Fig. 55. The difference in level between ears (a) for different directions of the sound source These are the averages from a number of experiments. The sources were about 1.5 meters away. The bottom graph (b) shows the amount of sound shadow at the far ear for different frequencies. (From Durlach and Colburn, 1978)

Most of our interest in understanding the auditory system as a sensory input, however, is in localization rather than lateralization. With that emphasis, the first realistic study of interest in localization of sound sources was performed by Stevens and Newman in 1936. They narrowed the situation in the same ways we have been considering; they kept the source in a plane at about the level of the subject's ears, they performed the experiment out of doors with the subject on an elevated platform to keep reflections to a minimum. Some indication of the pains taken by the experimenters to achieve these conditions can be inferred from the photograph in Fig. 56.

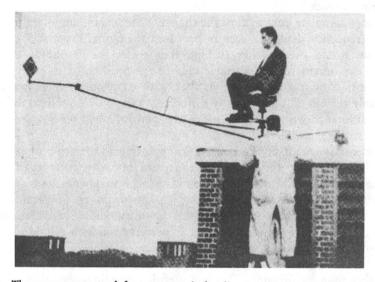

Fig. 56. The arrangement used for an open-air localization experiment. The small speaker swings in a full circle without giving any spurious sound clues. The roof of the building was 12 ft below the head of the listener. (From Stevens and Newman, 1936)

The procedure for the experiment was as follows: The sound source (a small loudspeaker) was placed for each trial at one of 13 positions spaced 15° apart, 0° being directly in front of the listener and 180° directly behind. The listener named the position he thought the tone came from. This was repeated, with position varying randomly from trial to trial, until each observer had made 10 judgments at each of the thirteen positions. Front back confusions (from any pair of comparable positions) were not counted as errors. We will look at this problem more closely later on. The tones varied in Sensation Level at different frequencies, but all were well above the background noise.

Relative size of localization error in this experiment for different frequencies is shown in (A) of Fig. 57. The results given for each frequency are averaged over all positions. The shape of the error curve is particularly intriguing following our discussion of the operation of time and intensity clues at low and high frequencies. It appears that as time difference begins to fail as an unambiguous clue there is a frequency region of slightly increased error before intensity ratio becomes a better clue at higher frequencies. Panel (B) of the figure indicates more precisely why we might predict the shape of

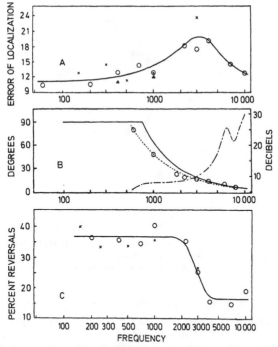

Fig. 57. *A* The relative number of localization errors at different frequencies. *B* The maximum angle that a tone is displaced from center by a change of 180° is shown by the solid curve. The circles show the actual maximum position change from 180° phase change. The dash-dot curve shows the intensity difference between ears when the sound is at one side. The drop in the error curve at high frequency may be due to the increasing usefulness of the intensity clue. *C* For low-frequency tones, front-back reversals are common. Above 3000 Hz the pinna probably furnishes some clue. (From Stevens and Newman, 1936)

the error curve. The solid line shows the location where our delay (*τ*) between ears is equal to half a period of the frequency on the base line; and the circles and dotted line show the maximum displacement for Halverson's (1927) listeners, using phase clues only (lateralization). At the right of panel (B) the dot-dash curve and the right-hand ordinate show the interaural intensity ratio for 90° azimuth. (Sivian and White, 1933.)

Why the large proportion of reversals at low frequencies as shown in panel (C) of Fig. 57? (40 % would mean complete indiscriminability.) A closer look at the geometry of source locations at the side of the head reveals that for any point close to a line through the two ears there is always an equidistant point on the other side of that line such that the distance between the two ears is the same as for the first point. If we extend our consideration outside the horizontal plane through the two ears, we can see in Fig. 58 that for a given *τ* between ears there is a large number of such points and they form a "cone of confusion" for that particular value of *τ*. A high degree of front-rear and up-down confusion should be expected if time between ears were the only clue. When the frequency of the sound is high enough that sound shadow is the mechanism, the lack of radial symmetry of the pinna probably helps.

One of the additional findings reported by Stevens and Newman is that

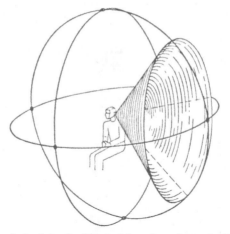

Fig. 58. A "cone of confusion" in the binaural location of sounds. From any point on the cone the delay between the two ears is essentially the same. The circles identify the three planes in which the sound can be specified

localization is finer at positions near the center than further toward the side. Later measurements that have used more closely spaced positions than 15° establish that, for lateralization studies, a displacement of 2° can be discriminated 75 % of the time at the midline position, but 7° is required for the same performance at 75° azimuth.

If we stopped our analysis at this point it might appear that location of sound sources is quite satisfactory and rather easily accounted for. But the several assumptions we made are not usually met, so the analysis is far from complete. Even in the limited domain of the horizontal plane we noted the prevalence of front-back confusions. These could be, and probably are, eliminated by slight rotations of the head.

We know from everyday observation that we also localize sound in the vertical dimension. Sound moving along an arc across the top of the head will produce time differences between ears of the same order as those we looked at in the horizontal plane. When do we respond to such changes as differences in height rather than in horizontal azimuth? The answer seems to be that we do so only when the sound contains frequencies with wavelengths comparable to the dimensions of the pinna. In experimenting on this aspect, Butler (1969) used bursts of noise to avoid the problem of the standing waves that are likely to be present whenever we use tones in the presence of any reflecting surface. Butler used some noises with high frequencies left in and some with high frequencies filtered out. Localization in the vertical plane was successful only when the signal contained frequencies in the neighborhood of 7 kHz and above. At these frequencies the wavelengths are a few centimeters and are of the order of the dimensions of the pinna.

The role of the pinna in localization has been a matter of some disagreement. Batteau (1968) felt that their shape gave them a special function. A simple analog of his formulation for localization by the pinna is the picket-fence acoustic effect. A sharp pressure wave traveling past a picket fence will create a separate pulse as it passes each aperture, and the observer hears a regular train of pulses. Batteau noted that the irregular shape of the pinna was such that pressure waves from a different angle would yield a different spacing of pulses from the irregular edges and promontories of the pinna. He postulated that these pulse transforms from different locations were internally stored for later identification of the angle of incidence (direction of arrival) of an impulse. Batteau made measurements on an enlarged model of the pinna that showed the changes in impulse transform shown in Fig. 59. One major problem is that, with regular size pinna, pulse-spacing changes of the order of 10—20 microseconds would have to be discriminated by the auditory analyzer. We saw in our discussion of time resolution that the system failed at spacings of 300—500 μsec with idealized pulses. This does not absolutely deny the possibility of learning much finer discriminations with experience but a reduction by a factor of 25 to 30 seems most unlikely.

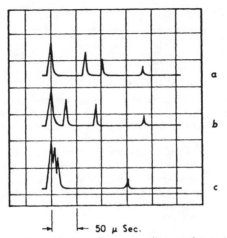

Fig. 59. Pulses synthesized from a microphone recording at the position of the eardrum in a simulated canal and pinna. These are the idealized pulse sequences from a single sharp pulse impinging on the irregularities of the pinna. When the pulse is from the front the sequence is as in *a*, *b* indicates the timing of pulses when the click comes from the side, and *c* from the rear. The simulated pinna and canal were 5 times normal size, so these must be scaled accordingly for the real ear. (From Batteau, 1968)

A puzzle remains, because a number of experiments (Batteau, 1967; Freedman and Fisher, 1968; Gardner and Gardner, 1973) indicate that not only is localization better with irregularly-shaped pinna, but possibly people localize more accurately with a mold of their own pinna on an artificial head than with a model of another person's pinna. The Gardner and Gardner experiment did not go that far. They used various attachments to accomplish different degrees of smoothing of the pinna of their listeners. Their signal was a broad band of noise, and it assumed positions in an arc extending above and below ear level in the frontal median plane. The results for different pinna "maskings" are shown in Fig. 60. We cannot as yet describe how it is accomplished, but it is experimentally well established that localization in the absence of head movement is better with a normally shaped pinna.

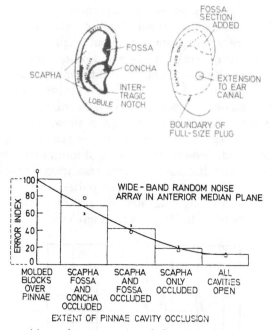

Fig. 60. The major cavities and promontories of the external ear are shown in the upper left. To the right are the outlines of the plugs used to smooth over these irregularities during the experiment. At the bottom is shown the effect of removing these plugs to restore the irregularities of the pinna. A score of 100 on the error index means the performance expected from pure guessing. These results are for a wide-band noise signal. Further work showed that the improvement can be attributed to high frequencies, the band from 8 to 10 kHz showing the most dramatic improvement. These results are for sounds from the front. For sounds from the rear the same phenomenon can be demonstrated, but the effects are smaller. (From Gardner and Gardner, 1973)

Interaural Time-Pattern Analysis

Time resolution of less than 100 microseconds may present problems for the monaural system. Not so for binaural perception. To get unequivocal estimates of the limit of interaural time resolution we need to deliver the signals by earphones, and thus we employ lateralization perceptions rather than localization. But it is our best estimate of the ultimate time resolution of the binaural system. Impulse signals are of greatest interest since these are the ones for which time differences are most apt to be useful. For a single click delivered to the two ears the time separation at the two ears must be 28 μsec before the observer can reliably tell which ear is lagging in time (Klumpp and Eady, 1956). For a longer train of pulses the required difference between ears is less.

We can take a burst of random noise to be the type of signal that has the properties of many natural signals of interest; it is essentially impulsive and constantly changing with time. Tobias and Zerlin (1959) used this signal to test the minimum time difference necessary to move perception of the signal off center and to see how the minimum necessary interaural delay changed as the signal lengthened. Their results show that for a noise burst as short as 10 msec the interaural delay must be 24 μsec. As the signal is made longer the necessary delay shortens until at 500 msec it requires only 6 or 7 μsec lead at one ear to move the signal just perceptibly off center. This is better precision than anyone has measured for true localization, since it would be the equivalent of movement of less than one degree off center. One thing that should be noted about these experiments is that each trial presents a centered burst along with the variable one. Our subjective memory of center is not good enough for this rather exceptional precision. How such infinitesimal intervals are preserved by a neural network whose units show a variability about 100 times as great as the minimum discernible interval is a matter of some puzzlement. We must conclude it is attributable to averaging out the error from a great many units.

So far all the signals we have considered have been single copies of a waveform to each ear. Seldom in everyday listening is the situation that simple. There are nearly always two or more reflecting boundaries near enough to give additional repetitions that will be above auditory threshold. Worse still, the position of the boundaries may be such that the lagging ear gets a reflection sooner than the leading ear. We still locate sounds with considerable success in such environments; in fact we also gain automatically an impression of some characteristics of the acoustic environment: size of enclosure, degree of reverberation, presence of single room resonance. The impression created by these characteristics is sometimes referred to as the acoustic coloration of the room.

Two auditory principles that aid in simplifying our sound perception in extremely complicated acoustic situations can be fairly easily sorted out. One we have already noted in assessing the time resolution of the system. This is the fusion of the original and the reflected duplicates of the waveform into a single perception. In reverberant environments the total pattern of reflections can be quite intricate, since sometimes all six boundaries may furnish at least one reflection, and there may be additional large reflecting objects in a room. For simplicity we can take the speed of sound to be about 1ft per millisecond, and we know that distances from walls, ceiling, etc. run several feet in the usual listening environment. For impulses in signal waveforms, then, the multiple-reflection pattern is theoretically aurally resolvable into separate pulses. It is fortunate indeed that the system fuses them into a single impression.

Recognition that a pattern of pulses should be fused is apparently related to duration of the pattern. From a number of experiments it appears that short patterns like single clicks are fused until the spacing is around 5—7 msec; for signals like continuous speech, the spacing may be 30—50 msec before the perception of a separate echo occurs.

The second principle that helps in unifying the perception of multiple reflections and probably prevents errors in some troublesome situations has several descriptive labels. It is known in America mostly as the precedence effect, in Europe it is the law of the first wave front, and it has also been called first-arrival effect and the auditory suppression effect. This conglomerate of names suggest how the effect operates: the direct wave from the source, which arrives first, is given more weight by the system than subsequent ones in judging what direction the sound came from.

We noted above that the position of source, listener and boundaries may be such that reflections may strongly suggest a false position for the source. Wallach, Newman and Rosenzweig (1949) set up a restricted click sequence under phones to test the relative efficacy of first and second interaural click pairs in determining the direction of the source. The time sequence for the two ears was that shown in Fig. 61. If the entire sequence takes place within about 2 msec we can be certain the listener will hear only one click because of the fusion effect discussed earlier. The single click heard will be on the side suggested by the first pair. But the suppression of the second pair is not complete, since whenever it is present the precision of subjective placement for the first pair goes down if the placement that would be suggested by the second pair by itself is different from that for the first.

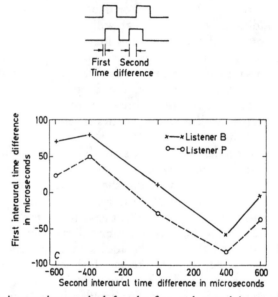

Fig. 61. The relative spacing required for the first and second interaural click to give a centered image. At the top is the time sequence of the clicks used, showing the placement of the first and second interaural time difference. The graph below shows how large the second interaural time difference must be to offset the first one and bring the single click image back to center. The implication is that the first image carries much greater weight in determining the location of an image. Of course, the antagonistic situation used in this experiment seldom occurs in normal sound localization. (From Wallach, Newman, and Rosenzweig, 1949)

Wallach, Newman and Rosenzweig made use of the fact that the second pair of clicks *does* have some influence on the first to get an estimate of the relative perceptual influence of the two. If they are set, as in the diagram, to suggest different directions, the influence of the second pair can be used to move the single fused click back to center. The results of Wallach, Newman and Rosenzweig indicate that if the click has been moved off center by a given delay, say 30 μsec, in the first pair, it takes 7 to 10 times as much opposing delay in the second pair to move the fused image back to center.

There are a number of reasons why we must suppose second clicks do not behave quite the same in normal listening environments. They are usually not of equal amplitude with the impulse from the original source, and probably have less influence than in the earphone experiment. They are also in general delayed by greater amounts. We have no clean comparisons of the precision of localization in reverberant and non-reverberant environments, but both extremely complicated acoustic situation can be fairly easily sorted out. experiment and everyday observation indicate that the law of the first wave front does operate.

Signal Selection by the Binaural System

Even from casual observation of our hearing behavior most of us connect the presence of two ears with our ability to locate sounds. The other function of binaural hearing we are apt to discover only in some circumstance when two-eared hearing fails to function. Koenig (1950) described a simple interesting maneuver for contrasting binaural hearing with monaural. In an environment where a number of people are talking simultaneously, such as a party, if the person speaking is just audible enough to be easily understood, closing one ear by inserting a finger will cause the voice being attended to become more difficult to hear and bring up the background voices noticeably.

This function of signal selection by the binaural system, like the study of lateralization rather than localization, can best be quantified in the laboratory under earphones. It has been studied using a variety of signals, but probably the most revealing demonstration is the following: A low-frequency pure tone in one earphone can be mixed with a noise in the same phone so that the tone is just barely audible, as we saw in our previous discussion of tonal masking by noise. If we now put exactly the same noise, but without the pure tone, into the opposite ear, the tone in the original ear becomes quiet clearly audible. Why has the introduction of noise in the opposite ear made the tone easier to hear? The answer is that it is not just any noise that we have added, but the same noise that is interfering with the tone. A simple analysis of the situation says that if we give the binaural analyzer a separate look at the noise, not mixed with the tone, it has a better technique for separating the tone from noise than when it only had the tone-noise mixture to work with. We can reinforce this impression further by adding the tone to the noise already in the second ear and seeing that the tone now is again almost inaudible. At first it may seem paradoxical that adding a tone has made the tone less audible, but the fact is that two looks as the same mixture of noise and tone is not as useful as a look at the sample of the noise separate from the noise-plus-tone mixture.

Another way to give the binaural system two different mixtures is to change the phase of the tone in one ear (with respect to the other ear). An easy way to do this, now that we have tone and noise in both ears with the tone scarcely audible, is to reverse the polarity of the tone in one ear. This would be the same as putting it 180° (π radians) out of phase. When this is done, the tone, which was barely audible with the noise and tone both in phase at the two ears, is quite easily heard. In fact, if we were to measure how much we can attenuate it to make it again just barely detectable it would require more than 10 dB of attenuation.

If it is true that those conditions where the tone is most clearly audible —given the same relative amounts of energy in signal (tone) and noise—are those that furnish two somewhat different mixtures of signal and noise at the two ears, then changing the phase at one ear by *less* than 180° should also improve the situation over the in-phase condition. It does, but by less than the 180° condition, *i.e.*, it does not require as much attenuation to render the tone again barely detectable.

Looking at this change of phase in one ear relative to the other as a time delay in one ear for the tone with no time delay for the interfering noise makes it apparent that there are some common elements with the conditions previously used for studying localization. Two different interaural delays not only would put the noise and tonal signal in two apparently different positions but would also, under some conditions make the signal more audible. How closely these two binaural phenomena of separation of sound sources in apparent space and enhancement of signal audibility through interaural differences are tied we do not yet know. They certainly have some elements in common.

Pure tones and white noise are not frequently encountered in everyday listening. But tones have the advantage of being easily specified and of occupying a single spot on the frequency dimension. White noise, on the other hand, is in some ways the ideal interfering signal, being continuously and evenly distributed over the frequency range. Consequently, for this phenomenon of binaural advantage in signal detection we have a gratifying wealth of data on the detection of tones in noise under various interaural conditions.

We have already looked at a comparison of some of these conditions in our illustrative example. A more complete list of conditions with their definitions is helpful and includes the following specifications of the signal and noise:

S_0 Signal presented to both ears; no interaural difference; image appears in center of head.

N_0 Noise presented to both ears; no interaural difference; noise image in center of head.

S_m Signal presented to one ear only; image at that ear.

N_m Noise presented to one ear only; noise image at that ear.

S_π Signal to both ears with waveform inverted at one ear; image at both ears or spread over a line between ears.

N_π Noise from same source to both ears but waveform inverted in one ear; image at both ears or extended on a line between ears.

N_u Noise at both ears but each ear from a different noise generator; image at the two ears.

S_τ Signal at both ears but delayed by τ time units at one ear; image lateralized toward the undelayed ear.

N_τ Noise at both ears but delayed at one ear; noise image lateralized toward undelayed ear.

S Signal at both ears but not in phase. This is a special case of S_τ.

With these shorthand designations we can list some interaural signal and noise combinations and their relative efficacy. The first step in the comparison is to specify a reference interaural condition. This could be designated $S_m N_m$, meaning that both noise and tone are in only one ear. This presupposes that detection of the tone in the noise is truly confined to the operation of only one ear[3]. Then the binaural advantage accruing to any other condition can be specified by measuring the difference in Sound Pressure Level of the signal when that signal is equally detectable in the noise under the two conditions. This difference is known as the Binaural Masking Level Difference (BMLD). Typical values for several interaural conditions are shown in Table 1. These are for a tone of 250 Hz, in the optimum frequency range for the BMLD.

Table 1. *The decibel advantage for various interaural relations of signal and noise*

Interaural Condition	BMLD (dB)
$N_o S_o$, $N_\pi S_\pi$, $N_u S_m$	0
$N_u S_\pi$	3
$N_u S_o$	4
$N_\pi S_m$	6
$N_o S_m$	9
$N_\pi S_o$	13
$N_o S_\pi$	15

Note that the three conditions in row 1 give no advantage over the monaural standard $N_m S_m$. Putting exactly the same signal and noise in both ears rather than one $(N_o S_o)$ does not make the signal more audible. Nor does it help to reverse polarity of *both* signal and noise in one ear $(N_\pi S_\pi)$; the system still gets only the same mixture of signal and noise. The fact that with an independent noise in the opposite ear the audibility of the signal in the test ear is not affected indicates that the system can recognize that that signal is unrelated and effectively exclude it. The other two entries with independent noise in the two ears $N_u S_\pi$ and $N_o S_u$ are slightly better than the standard, since the signal can be attenuated 3 to 4 dB to remain equally detectable. The 3 dB increase (amplitude ratio of $\sqrt{2} : 1$) is what we might predict from two independent analyzers under these same conditions.

The next two entries, $N_\pi S_m$ and $N_o S_m$ reinforce the impression in our original illustration that a look at the noise without the signal helps to separate

---

[3] If the noise introduced into the ear is not sufficiently stronger than the ambient noise in the two ears, the condition will not be truly monaural.

the two. The poorer performance when this separate look at the noise is inverted rather than identical might be predicted on the basis that a noise of opposite polarity in the two ears is never encountered in practice.

The last two conditions are the laboratory prototypes for BMLD for pure tones. To review the exact meaning: If we set a tone at a barely detectable level under the N_oS_o condition and simply reverse the polarity of the noise in one ear $(N_\pi S_o)$ the tone becomes so much more audible that it can be reduced 13 dB to be back at bare detectability again. Similarly for the 15 dB "gain" of the N_oS_π condition. This is a rather impressive performance for the binaural analyzer. 15 dB amounts to a reduction in amplitude of over 5 to 1. 5 to 1.

From what we have already seen of the gradual loss of time-pattern following as frequency is increased we could predict that at high frequencies inverting the waveform in one ear will no longer yield a binaural advantage. Experiments do show that the 15 dB advantage holds for low frequencies, tapers to about 6 dB at 1 kHz and to 3 dB at 1500 Hz.

The phenomenon is not confined to pure tones in noise. It has been shown also for tones masking tones, and noise masking noise as well. Of more general interest, if speech is set to where it is just detectable in interfering noise and then the speech waveform is inverted in one ear the speech can be attenuated by 12—13 dB before it is again just detectable (Levitt and Rabiner, 1967). Pulse trains masked by noise also show a BMLD when interaural conditions are changed from N_oS_o to N_uS_π. These can sound like a series of pulses at low rates (10—50 pps) or like steady-state complex tones at higher rates. Over the whole range of pulse rates, 10 pps to 1000 pps, over which Flanagan and Watson (1966) investigated BMLD for pulse trains N_oS_τ was more detectable than N_oS_o at the same S/N ratio. The greatest BMLD occurred for their 250 pps rate.

Flanagan and Watson also employed the N_oS_τ condition shown in our Table 1. They delayed the pulse train in one ear by varying amounts between 0 and 5 msec, and discovered that a delay of around 1.5 msec gave the highest BMLD. By employing filters to select the spectral content of their pulse trains and subjecting these filtered signals to different interaural time delays they concluded that signals with frequency content near 300 Hz *and* with an S_τ of about 1.5 msec (half the period of 300 Hz) contribute most to the BMLD. According to our frequency maps of the cochlea, this is quite close to the helicotrema. Presumably at this point binaural collating of neural impulses is optimum. This might also be concluded from the findings of Yost, Wightman and Green (1971) who showed that clicks with only low frequency information (500 Hz low-pass filtered) were more precisely lateralized (jnd $\approx$ 22 μsec) than clicks with only high-frequency information (above 2 kHz). The latter required a minimum interaural time difference almost 10 times as large. In the binaural processing of signals, there seems to be something special about the low frequency end of the membrane.

With the great bulk of this work on enhanced signal selection by the binaural system having been done under earphones, one may conjecture about how it relates to everyday hearing. It seems a bit anti-climactic that the most favorable interaural condition, S_π, would seldom, if ever, be realized outside the laboratory. However, the S_τ condition occurs whenever a sound source is located somewhere off the midline. Probably the most frequent condition is $N_\tau S_0$, since if listening is at all difficult we face the source of sound when possible. Not far behind would be $N_{\tau 1} S_{\tau 2}$ where both wanted and interfering sound came from locations off center, but not the same location. If they are on opposite sides of center we need to adopt a convention of designating right-leading as $+\tau$ and minus for left leading.

In hearing testing situations, where we attempt to measure the faintest sounds a subject or a patient can hear, these principles apply and definitely have their effect. We will return briefly to this topic when we define what we mean by normal hearing.

If we return to the noisy party environment where we first described the advantage of listening with two ears we can get a better notion why the contrast between monaural and binaural occurred. This acoustic situation has come to be known as the "cocktail party effect" since here we now have multiple possible sources at different azimuths to the listener. If we could make exact analogies, this might best fit the $N_u S_\tau$ designation, understanding that a special case occurs for S_0, when $\tau = 0$. Obviously, this is a great over-simplification, since the "noise" in this instance does not sound like an un-correlated mixture but rather like other voices, each with a different value of τ.

Switching from binaural to monaural and back in the cocktail party or similar situations makes the effect seem quite dramatic and seems to corrobo-rate the measured BMLD of 10 dB and better. However, if we attempt to measure the increase in *intelligibility* for speech, rather than simply the improved detection, the results are disappointing. The increase in intelligibility in the laboratory when we switch from $N_0 S_0$ to $N_0 S_\pi$ or to a favorable S_τ for speech is small. It is about the same increase in intelligibility that comes from increasing the speech gain by 3 or 4 dB in the presence of interfering noise. If we settle for only detecting the *presence* of the speech signal rather than measuring intelligibility, then the adventage is 12—13 dB for the best $(N_0 S_\pi)$ condition.

From the data we have thus far, we have to conclude that the BMLD is mostly a detection phenomenon. How much better other processing operations are accomplished binaurally than monaurally must await more complete measures.

Part III
Hearing Loss

Thus far we have been pursuing an understanding of the operation of the normally-functioning auditory system. It should be apparent that it is a fairly intricate system. Despite our incomplete understanding of its function, we have ample empirical evidence that it does perform even in the face of fairly severe distortion of familiar signals. Indeed, it would be fair to say that the normally-operating system is unusually robust in its resistance to the effects of distortion.

This adaptability of the processing system may also mean that minor malfunctions can occur and go unnoticed. But we also know from acquaintance with the hearing-impaired population that major malfunctions of the system do occur, and that they interfere to a distressing degree with the reception of speech and meaningful environmental sounds. Such partial failures of the system—short of total deafness—are referred to by the generic term hearing loss. In diagnosing the nature of the disorder and in predicting the likelihood of remediation it is of paramount importance to understand the changes that take place when the auditory system fails to function properly.

We have been reviewing the mechanisms that serve to explain what we know of the processing of auditory signals. Much of the attempt to understand dysfunction of the system centers on the possible failure of these mechanisms.

It is advisable to remember that this amounts to a sort of second order of uncertainty, since the original details of the postulated processing mechanisms have been established mostly by inference. But the collating of information from audiology, psychoacoustics and auditory neurophysiology has already been of tangible help in elucidating some of the behavior of auditory systems that do not function normally. The major precaution needed is that explanations must remain flexible in keeping with the incompleteness of our understanding.

Is the fault simply that the system is no longer sensitive enough to pick up the usual signals of the environment? If so, mechanical repair may be possible, as we shall see in our discussion of conductive hearing loss. In spite of the fact that we must deal with such unbelievably small amplitudes of movement, we have a fair understanding of the mechanical operation of the system—at least through the middle ear where mechanical malfunction is most likely to be found.

For other types of system failure we look for differences in those aspects that our engineering models have led us to believe are indispensable to auditory signal processing. In this vein a number of interesting possibilities have been explored for understanding the nature of departures from normal function. Since spectral analysis has seemed to play a fundamental role in auditory processing, one notion is that the filter-like mechanisms no longer function normally. This question may take the form of asking whether the critical bandwidths are different in certain kinds of hearing loss than in normal ears.

Actually, this question has been explored in two interesting ways. Both critical ratios and critical bands have been measured in patients with non-conductive (sensorineural) loss. Though the results are highly variable from patient to patient, in general they do imply poorer spectral resolution. Secondly, analogous measurements of neural tuning have been performed in cats with cochleas that have been subjected to some of the same agents suspected of contributing to dysfunction. Some of these have been hypoxia, blocking of cochlear blood supply, ototoxic drugs or diffusion of contaminated or diseased perilymph into the cochlea to be analyzed. Since there is reason to suppose that some of the tuning that takes place in the cochlea is accomplished after the mechanical tuning the expectation is that measurement of nerves from these cochleas will show wider response areas than normal. This supposition is borne out by the data (Evans, 1978).

What seems to prevail is the belief that the normal temporal and spectral (lateral?) suppression mechanisms are lacking or faulty and that therefore the effective auditory signal-to-noise ratio is poorer for ears with sensorineural loss. How much of the analysis and separation of signals we know to be accomplished by the system is dependent on the tuning that takes place in the cochlea is not directly traceable, but it seems axiomatic that breakdown of cochlear tuning would contribute to faulty later analysis.

Conductive Loss 12

Normal Hearing Standards

In considering the sensitivity of the ear, we made use of a pair of curves by Sivian and White showing the minimum audible sound levels at different frequencies. These have been the standard "threshold" curves for much of auditory work for the decades since. It can hardly be claimed, however, that they represent a formal standard for normal pure-tone thresholds. They were taken on 9 people at the Bell Laboratories who presumably had normal hearing, but were selected mostly for convenience. The measurements were taken in an acoustic environment that is ideal for measuring absolute sensitivity, but not easy to duplicate—namely a well isolated, anechoic chamber. When we prepare to work with or to understand auditory systems that are not functioning normally different considerations apply in setting a baseline for normal hearing for pure tones.

As soon as tuning forks for testing hearing began to be replaced by audiometers, the question of a standard for zero hearing loss arose. Two major questions ought to be settled. (1) How does one select a representative sample, and what statistic from that sample is the appropriate one for Zero on the Hearing Loss scale? (2) How should the physical standard be specified so it can be duplicated at different places?

In America, a number of large samples were tested, starting with a compilation of audiograms by the Public Health Service in 1938; then a large sample at the World's Fair in 1939, volunteers at the San Diego County Fair in 1950 and the Wisconsin State Fair in 1954. The first standard, set by the American Standards Association in 1951, drew heavily on such group measurement. Experience with that standard, improvement in audiometric technique, and some valuable experience in transferring results from one laboratory or group to another led to international standardization in 1964, by the International Standards Organization (ISO, 1964). Many American audiometer manufacturers and clinics currently employ a later standard by the American National Standards Institute (ANSI, 1969), but the two differ negligibly for pure tone threshold measurement.

A brief look at the problems posed by point (2) is warranted. In just what form do we specify the value for audiometric zero? In their measure of the sensitivity curve, Sivian and White (see Chap. 6) spoke of minimum audible field as the SPL measured by a microphone at the position of the listener's head, and minimum audible pressure as the sound pressure at the eardrum. This latter was measured with a phone on the ear, and a slim probe inserted in the ear canal measured the sound pressure at the eardrum. This is an intricate measurement and not practical for duplicating standards at the many installations that require a calibrated standard for audiometric measurement.

What is done instead is to measure the Sound Pressure Level developed in a standard coupler with the same electrical input to the phone. Actually since the electrical input to the phone is so small at auditory threshold, the measurement is usually made 60 dB above and the threshold level is calculated on the assumption the system is linear.

That particular procedure is not confined to standardizing measurements for auditory threshold. Many measurements of performance of the ear are necessarily made with earphones. Hence it is necessary to have a calibrating device to substitute for the ear to check the stability of the equipment and to duplicate the results of such measurement. Because these devices have been used as this kind of calibrating substitute for the ear, they have sometimes been called "artificial ears". In most instances, however, the device used is simply a 6 cc coupler of specified dimensions. Such devices ought properly to be designated as calibrating couplers, and the term artificial ear reserved for devices designed to imitate much more closely the characteristics of the ear. One such device developed by Zwislocki employs six separate cavities to imitate various aspects of the acoustic auditory system.

The fact that the standard 6 cc coupler is only a rough analog of the acoustic load the ear presents to the phone makes one additional problem. If we wish to use a new type of phone it is not enough to require that the new phone produces the same SPL into the coupler microphone. Producing the same level in the coupler does not mean the same threshold levels. In general, the phone will interact differently with the coupler than it does with the ear. It would be awkward, however, to repeat the whole standardization with each new phone. Fortunately, the appropriate procedure is to compare the performance of the new phone with the old on the ear itself, specifically by a loudness match. If it takes x dB more (or less) SPL for the new phone to create an equally loud signal in the ear it also requires the same difference to create zero loudness (threshold). The final step in the transfer of standard to a new phone is to put the new phone on the standard coupler with 60 dB less attenuation than was required for threshold. The new standard is the SPL read on the coupler microphone.

Coupler measurement is thus the method for specifying and duplicating auditory signal levels and especially for calibrating clinical audiometers.

Reference threshold sound pressure levels for pure tone audiometers are shown in Fig. 62 and they differ little from the curve from the Sivian and White minimum audible pressure measurements. These are also very close to the values adopted by the American National Standards Institute (ANSI) in 1969. Watson and his colleagues (Watson *et al.*, 1972) conducted some very careful laboratory measurements of the detection of pure tones at audiometric frequencies in a very quiet environment. Their levels for 50—75 % detectability lie reassuringly close to the ANSI recommendations. They also concluded that at these levels "system noise" of the individual was the probable limiting factor.

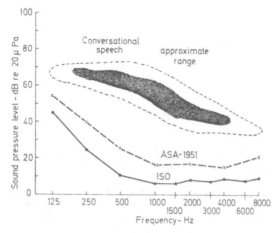

Fig. 62. Pure tone Sound Pressure Levels for audiometric zero. Most audiometers are calibrated so that the SPL designated by the dots and the solid line is the level produced in a standard 6 cc coupler from the audiometer phone when the audiometer dial is set to zero. These were adopted by the International Standards Organization in 1964. For historical interest the values recommended by the American Standards Association in 1951 are included. The area of the speech sounds is included for comparison of the shape and the slope of the speech area with the audiometric zero curve. The vertical placement of the speech area is arbitrary. (Modified from Davis and Silverman, 1978)

But what is the practical significance of audiometric zero? We seldom listen at those levels, partly because in most environments ambient noise lies well above audiometric zero, and because in any event we prefer speech signals comfortably above our threshold. Departures of 10—15 dB from normal audiometric threshold are not taken as signs of present hearing difficulty but as possible warnings that future tests should be scheduled to see whether such a departure from zero dB indicates a trend or only a temporary anomalous loss of sensitivity.

Tests for Conductive Loss–The Audiogram

Audiologists and otologists prefer not to be concerned with the actual physical shape of the pure tone threshold. They use instead a graph like that shown in Fig. 63. When an audiometer has been calibrated for pure tone

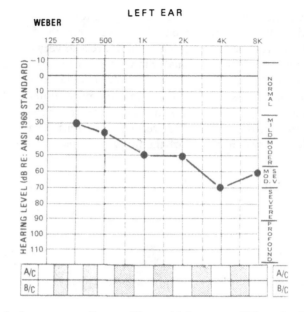

Fig. 63. A standard pure tone audiogram. The sensitivity curve of Fig. 62 has been straightened by defining 0 dB Hearing Level on this graph as equal at any frequency to the Sound Pressure Level on that standard "threshold" curve. Thus two tones at 250 Hz and 500 Hz might both be at 10 dB Hearing Level, but they would differ by 15 dB in Sound Pressure Level. A patient whose pure tone hearing measured as shown by the circles would be said to have a mild-to-moderate loss in the low frequencies and a moderate-to-moderately-severe loss in the high frequencies

testing and its Hearing Level dial is set at zero, the sound pressure level that the audiometer phone creates in a standard 6 cc coupler should be that shown in Fig. 62 for any of the standard frequencies. Here we have a slightly different use of the decibel scale: Zero dB on the Hearing Level scale is that sound pressure level designated as standard reference threshold by the ANSI specification. A tone with 10 times the intensity of the standard has a Hearing Level of 10 dB, etc. A person who is tested on the audiometer and fails to hear tones lower than 40 dB on the Hearing Level dial has a Hearing Threshold Level (HTL) of 40 dB.

Testing a patient's hearing for pure tones gives only part of the information needed for assessment of a hearing loss, but it is a very important part. It can indicate the shape and the severity of the loss over the important part of the frequency range. Recommended technique is to present tones of a second or so in length and to have the listener (patient) indicate when he hears the tone. This may be by pressing a button or by raising a finger while the tone is on. The tester starts well above the suspected threshold and gradually attenuates the tone until a level is found where the patient responds correctly about half the time. This is done for each of the standard audiometric frequencies: 125, 250, 500, 1000, 2000, 4000 and 8000 Hz. On some audiometers the intermediate frequencies of 750, 1500, 3000, and 6000 Hz are also included.

Possibly the most easily understood reason for a patient not to show normal hearing sensitivity is some failure of the mechanical part of the ear. But many other factors can contribute to a departure from normal sensitivity, so it is desirable to know whether mechanical failure is the underlying cause. In the language commonly adopted, we want to know whether this is a conductive loss.

One way of testing whether the loss is conductive has been to reason that most mechanical failures would involve the canal and middle ear structures. If we could vibrate the fluid in the cochlea without transmitting sound through the outer and middle ear we could narrow down the locus of the difficulty. This is the rationale of testing hearing by bone conduction. A bone vibrator is placed on the skull, either on the mastoid bone or on the forehead, depending on which way the audiometer has been calibrated, and the patient's hearing for bone-conducted sound is measured by the same procedures as described for air conducted sound. As implied, standard levels for bone conduction stimulation have also been agreed upon. These are not a subject of universal agreement at this date (1979), but most clinics have a workable method for calibration which we will discuss later on.

A look at the principles of bone-conducted stimulation of the cochlea should be very useful. For our present purposes the vastly simplified diagram of Fig. 64 should suffice. The "volume" enclosed by the heavy line represents the fluid encased in the cochlea, the spring is the combined flexibility of the eardrum, ligaments and muscles of the middle-ear structures. Similarly the attached mass is the combined mass of all the movable middle ear structures.

If we simplify correspondingly the action of a vibrator on the skull, it can be considered to have two different effects. If it moves the skull bodily back and forth, the entire encased fluid will be moved with the surrounding skull, but the spring and mass combination is not attached rigidly and will tend to move with a phase and amplitude different from the fluid. The effect is to move the piston (stapes) in the oval window in a fashion similar to that for air conducted sound. This component is referred to as inertial bone conduction. It will be the dominant component of bone conduction at low frequencies.

The other action of the vibrator on the head is to create compressional waves. They may occur because of compressional waves spreading through

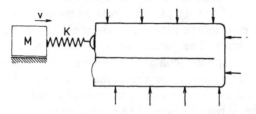

Fig. 64. A simple hydromechanical analog of hearing by bone conduction. If the stapes is rigidly locked in the oval window, the spring and mass of the middle ear components will have little effect. All the yielding will be done at the round window. This yielding will still result in a pressure difference between the two scala and subsequent motion of the membrane

the relatively homogeneous (acoustically) tissue, fluid and bone of the head, or they may result from flexural waves traveling on the bony casing. In either case the result of interest is alternate compression and rarefaction of the bone surrounding the cochlear labyrinth. This is indicated by the arrows suggesting the action on the cochlea during the compression phase. The result of this action is governed by the same Pascal's principle that we invoked to understand normal air conduction. In this instance the principle is applied in reverse, since here a pressure at all points on the boundary of the container will be transmitted to the two windows—one closed by the stapes and one by the round window membrane. So long as these two windows respond differently, either in amplitude or phase, to the pressure of the fluid, the conditions for the generation of the traveling wave down the basilar membrane are essentially the same as in air conduction.

Even from this simplified model for bone-conducted stimulation of the cochlea, it is apparent that the old notion that bone conduction completely bypasses the middle ear structures is not tenable. What is fortunate for clinical testing is that ears with conductive loss show roughly the same sensitivity by bone conduction as normal ears, even though the detailed mode of response may differ. This does not mean, of course, that the bone-conduction sensitivity curve looks anything like the air-conduction curve, or that sensitivity for the two modes is equal in any demonstrable sense. Discrepancies in the energy required by the two modes of stimulation are compensated in the calibration of the audiometer so that a setting of zero on the Hearing Level dial furnishes the appropriate energy for whichever output transducer is switched in. Standards for calibration of bone conduction by an artificial mastoid, of similar purpose as the 6 cc coupler for air conduction, is under consideration by standards groups.

However it comes about, changes in the conducting mechanism of the ear do not generally change significantly its magnitude of response to bone-conducted sound, and this makes the bone conduction pure tone test a very useful diagnostic tool. Since inner ear and neural losses must affect both air and bone tests equally, only rarely does an ear with a loss show greater pure tone sensitivity by air conduction than by bone. Hence, in testing any patient, the departure of the bone conduction results from zero dB HL can quite safely be taken as an estimate of the amount of non-conductive loss.

Thus far we have been discussing pure tone testing without much awareness of its difficulties. For very practical reasons we need to assess the performance of the two ears independently. Even with air conduction testing this may present a problem. The patient wears a phone that must be in contact with the head. The phone contains a moving element that is bound to transmit some of its vibration to the pinna; and even the vibration of the air against the walls of the canal must contribute to vibration of the head. If this seems unlikely, it may be helpful to remember that we saw in our investigation of the sensitivity of the ear that movements of the order of less than an Ångstrom are sufficient to lead to a sensation of hearing in the normal ear. How much of this gets to the opposite ear in the form of bone conducted sound? This is an important question, since we *do* need to test the two ears independently, and if sound at the non-test ear is only x dB down from sound at the test ear, then we cannot test the bad ear when it is x dB (or more) less sensitive than the good ear.

The way around this difficulty is to use another sound to mask the better ear when testing the poorer one. This requires that we test the better ear first, or at least that we know its pure-tone thresholds when testing the poorer ear. Since we saw that the leakage to the opposite ear may well be by bone conduction, and since we know that the bone conduction threshold will be as good as or better (lower) than air conduction, we adopt the rule that if the non-test ear has a bone conduction threshold x dB or more better than the test ear we need to add a steady masking noise in the better ear.

Finding the value of x dB is an empirical matter. The situation is too complex and too variable for precise analysis. In the actual testing situation, in addition to the leakage paths already mentioned, the phone cushions may not seal well enough and that air-leakage path may contribute. The head-band may also help to transmit vibration. Overall, with the headsets currently in use, a workable rule is that if the threshold of the non-test ear is better than the test ear by 35 dB, masking should be used in the better ear.

For bone conduction, the problem of ear independence is much greater. Considering the possibility of flexural waves in the skull and of translational movement of the head (remembering how small these amplitudes can be) there is no guarantee that even for placement of the bone vibrator behind the test ear the amplitude will be any smaller at the opposite ear. Consequently, when there is any reason to suspect any difference in bone conduction sensitivity at the two ears, the non-test ear should be masked. For efficiency in the sense of having the masking noise be no louder or annoying than it need be to do the job, and also for the sake of not stimulating unnecessarily other segments of the basilar membrane that are to be tested later, the masking sound on most audiometers is a band of noise about the width of one critical band at the frequency of the test tone.

Sensitivity for pure tones represented at one time most of the information gathered on patients in the audiology clinic and the otologist's office. This is no longer the case, but the pure tone audiogram is still done routinely on most patients. An illustrative result is shown in Fig. 63.

Tympanometry

With advances in instrumentation, the notion arose that any significant change in the conductive mechanism of the ear could be measured as a change of impedance at the eardrum. Impedance in general means the amount of opposition offered to an oscillating driving force. In the case of the ear the oscillatory driving force is the sound wave in the air. Impedance measurement is highly developed for the testing of other acoustic materials and devices. It involves furnishing a calibrated driving wave to the device and measuring the amplitude and phase of the reflected wave. Impedance of a complex device like the mechanical auditory system is not a simple concept. For a simple mechanical (including acoustical) device the formula is

$$Z_m = \left[R^2 + \left(2_\pi f M - \frac{S}{2_\pi f} \right)^2 \right]^{1/2}$$

where R = frictional resistance

$2_\pi f M$ = mass reactance

$\dfrac{S}{2_\pi f}$ = stiffness reactance

$2_\pi f$ = frequency in radians

It can be seen that impedance is a complex quantity (real + imaginary). For many purposes the expression can be reduced to

$$Z_m = R + jX, \text{ with } X = 2_\pi f M - \frac{S}{2_\pi f}.$$

In such instances, measurement of the magnitude and the angle of the reflected wave will suffice for each frequency needed. But even with this simplification, a complete measure of ear impedance over the frequency range of interest is not easy to accomplish. Zwislocki (1957, 1963) brought the concept to a fairly high stage of development with his measurement of impedance of both normal and pathological ears but, even with techniques too advanced for the clinic, most of Zwislocki's measurements were confined to frequencies below 1 kHz. Attempts in America to take the technique into the audiology clinic have been partly successful at a few places, but the majority of clinics, though they may use the terminology of impedance measurement are using a modified impedance bridge and a single input frequency around 200 Hz (sometimes 660 Hz also) to measure primarily the mobility of the mechanical auditory system. Mobility is intended in the common-sense meaning but the translation of the term to the formal terminology of impedance is almost automatic because the reciprocal of stiffness (see above) is compliance, measured in cc of volume. Now at low frequencies, the mechanical auditory system has negligible resistance and mass reactance compared to its stiffness reactance, so that if we measure its compliance (1/stiffness) we have essentially measured its mobility, which is the reciprocal of impedance.

The very useful clinical extension of this simplification of impedance measurement has been the development of the technique of tympanometry. The principle involved is that the compliance or mobility of the mechanical system will be greatest when it is not stressed by a static difference in pressure on the two sides of the eardrum. The apparatus for tympanometry is shown in Fig. 65. A simplified form of the impedance bridge is used to plot the system mobility as the pressure in the ear canal is changed from +200 mm H₂O to — 300 mm H₂O.

The principle is quite a simple one. A standard tone of 220 Hz at a calibrated level is fed into the ear canal. The amount reflected back to the microphone will depend on the compliance of the cavity; the more compliant,

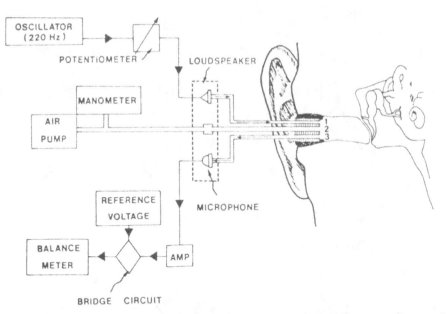

Fig. 65. Block diagram of the usual scheme for measuring the mobility (compliance) of the middle ear mechanism. What is actually measured is the loudspeaker driving voltage necessary to create enough level in the ear canal to make the microphone voltage match the reference voltage. This is related to how much sound was reflected rather than transmitted through the middle ear. The manometer and pump create the desired static pressure difference between ear canal and middle ear. The less mobile the drum, the less its action is affected by the static pressure difference. (See text)

the less reflection, other things being equal. First of all, consider the normal mechanism. If the mechanical system is stressed by having normal atmospheric pressure in the middle ear, but —200 mm H_2O pressure in the canal the compliance will be less than normal. As the canal pressure is returned to normal the pressure differential across the drum is less and the compliance rises. As the canal pressure is taken past normal to a positive pressure, compliance again gets less because the system is stressed in the opposite direction. A plot of the resulting relative compliance values for mechanically normal ears will fall inside the shaded area of the graphs in Fig. 66. Actually, even in normal middle ears the peak compliance may be reached when the pressure is about 50 mm H_2O less than normal. This happens because the oxygen in the trapped air in the middle ear gets gradually absorbed creating a slightly lower than normal pressure. Until the Eustachian tube opens to equalize this pressure the system is least stressed (most compliant) when the ear canal pressure is also slightly negative. When for any reason the Eustachian tube remains closed, the plot of changing compliance with changing pressure will look like type C of the figure. It is diagnostically important that it occurs with serous otitis media, but early acute otitis media may show a positive middle ear pressure.

The tracing labeled Type A_D in the Figure shows what occurs when the compliance changes much more than normal as the pressure is varied. The

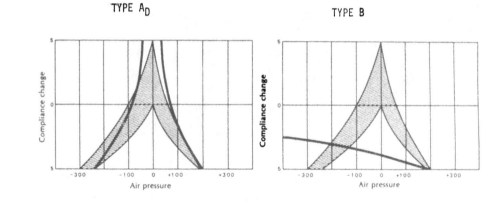

TYPE A_D

TYPE B

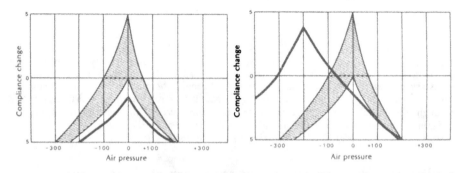

TYPE A_S

TYPE C

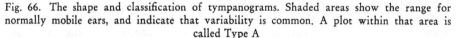

Fig. 66. The shape and classification of tympanograms. Shaded areas show the range for normally mobile ears, and indicate that variability is common. A plot within that area is called Type A

Type A_D: This is most apt to occur when the ossicular chain is interrupted or when the drum is too flaccid

Type A_S: This pattern results when the drum is less mobile than normal. Somewhere along the mechanical transmission chain a fixation has occurred

Type B: This pattern is indicative of fluid in the middle ear. Pulling the drum outward (negative pressure) makes it move a little easier

Type C: From negative pressure in the middle ear. The Eustachian tube is blocked and not equalizing the pressure

subscript, *D*, is for deep, though possibly *P* for peaked would be more descriptive. This happens when the drum is not attached firmly to the rest of the system—a discontinuity of the ossicular chain—or when the drum itself is less structurally rigid than normal. Ossicular discontinuities can occur with repeated invasion from middle ear disease or from a traumatic impact. In either of these cases the drum no longer drives the rest of the system as efficiently as usual.

If, on the other hand, the mechanical transmission system is rigidly attached at some point, the tracing will resemble Type *A_s* (shallow). This can occur with fixation of the ossicular chain to the bony wall at some point, as with otosclerosis or adhesions associated with serous otitis media or middle ear tumors. The system still shows some change in compliance from stressing by air pressure difference—except in cases of extremely rigid fixation—but it is inherently too rigid to be significantly affected by the differential pressure changes of tympanometry.

If the middle ear is filled with fluid or some other substance than air, then the change in compliance will look like Type *B* in the Figure. Serous otitis media or middle-ear tumor might give rise to this configuration. This can be a serious problem in children. Some idea of what happens in the middle ear can be gained from a look at Fig. 67, which shows the difference in the normal middle ear and one with purulent otitis media. Not only is the drum thickened, but there is almost no compliant cavity behind it. Repeated episodes can lead to erosion of the ossicular chain in some instances or to fixation to the middle ear wall in others. Tympanometry is of inestimable assistance in detecting middle ear congestion long before it reaches this stage.

Two other tests related to the mechanical operation of the system are made with the same apparatus shown in Fig. 65. The equivalent volume of the middle ear is of some supplementary diagnostic use, and is easily computed from essentially the same tympanometric measures we haven been following. When the eardrum and the rest of the mechanical system are stressed by a large positive pressure (200 mm H_2O) in the canal, the drum acts as a reflecting boundary with the result that the compliance measured (in cc) is essentially that volume in front of the drum, namely the unfilled part of the ear canal (see Fig. 65). At the pressure yielding maximum compliance, usually when the pressure on the two sides of the drum is equal, the measured compliance is that of the entire system, including the canal. Thus subtracting the stressed measure from the unstressed yields the compliance of the system minus the canal, and this is taken to be the equivalent volume of the middle ear cavity. In normally operating ears, this measure varies widely—from 0.28 cc to 1.25 cc—overlapping widely with values from clinical ears.

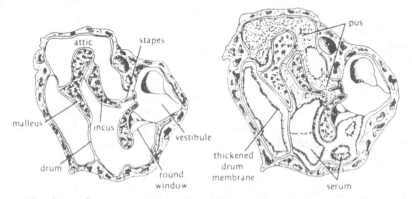

Fig. 67. The shape of a cross section of the middle ear through the center of the ossicular chain. The acoustic effect of the presence of fluid from middle-ear disease can be deduced from the drawing on the right. Increased production of fluid can make the pressure great enough to rupture the eardrum. This condition would yield a Type B tympanogram. (From Davis and Silverman, 1978)

One instance when the equivalent volume measure is definitely useful is the case of a perforation in the drum. Even when these are too small to be easily visible, the low frequency of the test sees the two cavities as one and the equivalent compliance is abnormally large.

It might be of at least passing interest to note that even when the system is stressed with a pressure differential of 200 mm H₂O the structures of the ear are displaced very little. Békésy's measurements on human ears indicate that with a varying pressure of 10^3 dynes/cm² (134 dB SPL) the stapes would move only 0.2 micron at low frequencies. (Békésy, 1960, p. 173.) If only a very rough estimate will suffice this can be likened to a pressure of 10 mm H₂O, so a 200 mm H₂O pressure might move the structures as much as 4 microns. Displacements of this order from sounds in the audible range are dangerous, but static displacements of the same magnitude are not even uncomfortable. The elastic parts of the drum may of course show larger displacement when stressed.

The second easily available measure using the same equipment is the middle ear muscle reflex. Just as we can stress the mechanical system by applying pressure in the canal, the stapedius muscle will act to restrain the movement of the ossicular chain with much the same effect. Measurement of the lowest level of sound for which the acoustic reflex occurs is of use in assessing the existence of the reflex and can be an additional check on the adequacy of the mechanical system.

The most frequently used technique takes advantage of the fact that the reflex is bilateral, that is, if it is elicited by a signal in either ear the muscles on both sides will contract. With the Balance Meter of Fig. 65 at center, a tone or a noise is introduced into the opposite ear. When the tone is strong enough to elicit the reflex, the amount of sound reflected to the microphone will increase giving an indication of increased impedance on the balance meter.

Normal ears require a pure tone Hearing Level of about 85 dB to elicit the reflex, or a broad band noise will lead to a contraction at about 65 dB HL (Deutsch, 1972). If a signal at the appropriate level fails to show a meter deflection this is presumptive evidence of either a loss in the ear with the signal, an absence of the reflex contraction, or a failure of the contraction to show because of a mechanical rigidity in the ear where the measurement is being made. If the ear with the test signal has a conductive loss of x dB at some frequency, then the reflex should show at $(85 + x)$ dB HL at that frequency. For a sensorineural (non-conductive) loss the situation is more complicated and we will discuss it when we know more about that kind of loss. The usefulness of the reflex threshold as a measure of loss is greatest in those situations where the patient does not respond voluntarily, for example with very young children.

In areas where medical attention is easily available, permanent conductive losses are not nearly as common as they once were. This is not true for secretory otitis media in young children. Even more cases than previously of middle ear involvement seem to appear in recent years (Ginsberg and White, 1978), possibly because of better recognition of the problem. But with proper attention, these need not lead to permanent problems in the middle ear. Even a congested middle ear can usually be cleared with decongestants and with ventilating tubes and will return to normal mechanical operation.

The mechanical auditory system is an admirable device which continues to function for years without signs of wear. On the other hand, it is subject to a number of mechanical malfunctions of varying degree of severity. The external canal can become blocked or partially blocked, usually by cerumen. Fluid may accumulate in the middle ear, sometimes from allergy or respiratory infection. As seen in Fig. 67, this has a definite effect on the acoustics of the drum and the middle-ear cavity. A perforation of the drum, even a very small one, will have its effect on the transmission curve of the middle ear by obviating the required pressure differential across the drum, but will also increase the likelihood of middle-ear infection. Bony or fibrous fixation of points on the suspension of the middle-ear structures (see Fig. 5) can interfere with mobility of the structures. Either mechanical trauma, such as a severe head blow, or necrosis or atrophy of the thin portion of the incus can cause a discontinuity at the juncture of the incus and stapes.

But though the otologist sees many of these, the probability of occurrence in the population is small. Most of the losses accompanying aging show very little conductive component. When mechanical losses do occur at an early age, medical repair of the middle-ear structures is growing more and more successful. Microsurgery of the middle ear may take the form of simply freeing the stapes footplate if it has become partially "frozen" by the bone growth of otosclerosis. It may also, however, require substituting a new footplate if the stapes must be removed, or a replacement for all or some part of the ossicular chain. This may mean that the new connection between ossicular chain and inner ear fluid is a wire or a tantalum strut resting against a new footplate of cartilage. Failing that, amplification through a hearing aid is a successful remedy for all except the very severe conductive losses.

13 Cochlear Dysfunction

Most patients who come to the audiology clinic or the doctor's office know only that they do not hear the things other people hear. Whether this happens because of failure of the mechanical part of the auditory system, something amiss in the cochlea or some problem with the neural components of the system is a problem for the otologist or the audiologist.

We have just seen that a number of clinical tools assist in the identification of conductive *vs* non-conductive loss. If there is a loss by air conduction but not by bone conduction, if the middle ear shows either little change in mobility or far too much change with differences in air pressure across the drum, and if middle ear muscle reflexes do not occur until abnormally high signal levels are reached, there can be little doubt that the mechanical part of the system is at fault. But if the system shows normal mobility, the pure-tone sensitivity loss is the same by air and by bone conduction, and the muscle reflex threshold is shifted, but not necessarily by the amount of the loss, then the problem is to decide whether it is an inner ear dysfunction or something beyond the cochlea.

The cochlea represents the first stage of processing of sound in the auditory system. We have already seen that it is a highly specialized end organ and a very sensitive one. Even electrically, one can scarcely any longer regard the cochlea as analogous to a passive device like the crystal microphone; it resembles instead a battery-powered active set of elements which make it possible to operate on far less input energy than would otherwise be the case (Thalmann, 1975). It follows that it also contains some very vulnerable structures—particularly the sensitive hair cells whose function is to transduce the sound from mechanical to neural or electrochemical form. The high metabolism of the cochlea makes it susceptible to agents in the bloodstream such as drugs. The highly deleterious effect of the mycins are now well publicized so that they are used mostly only for life-saving procedures. Aspirin and quinine are known to cause temporary loss of sensitivity, but there is no evidence of irreversible damage from these agents. Diuretics appear to have a deleterious effect. Periods of anoxia certainly have a temporary effect; at what point it becomes irreversible is not established. Any bacterial infection invading the perilymph poses a threat to the inner ear. Exposure to noise, whether it be a very high-level traumatic exposure or continued exposure at sub-traumatic levels leads to permanent loss. This is discussed at greater length in connection with temporary and permanent threshold shift.

One or more of these risks to well-being of the inner ear will inevitably occur one or more times during any individual's life, and it may be that this is sufficient to account for the loss with old age, called presbycusis. There may also be a small conductive component associated with additional ossification and the stiffening of ligatures and tendons, but this has been suspected only in very advanced age. The primary symptoms of presbycusis are those we will find associated with cochlear dysfunction. A good idea of the extent of this change in hearing sensitivity with age is gained from the portrayal in Fig. 68. This shows sensitivity loss for pure tones only. Most persons with presbycusis have in addition the other problems that we will note in describing cochlear dysfunction, such as undue trouble understanding speech and much difficulty listening in environments with other interfering signals.

With this sample of near-clinical, age-related losses added to the other persons with inner ear losses who come to the doctor's office and the clinic, cochlear dysfunction is by far the most common class of hearing disorder. One vexing problem in attempting to establish the nature of inner ear dysfunction is that the operating cochlea cannot be observed visually, even with our best technical aids.

The first task, then, for the audiologist is to establish the extent of non-conductive loss at each audiometric frequency. If tympanometry or muscle reflex measurements have indicated that there is some conductive component, then the initial focus may be on how much the bone conduction threshold departs from normal. The *additional* loss by air conduction—the air-bone gap—may need to be weighed separately for it may respond to remedial procedures, whereas the non-conductive loss likely will not.

Békésy Audiograms

With an indication that there is at least some sensorineural (non-conductive) component to the loss, a number of additional tests are advisable. Possibly the most efficient of these is the Békésy threshold-tracing test. The Békésy audiometer consists of a tone source that changes frequency at a fixed rate and an attenuator that changes the amplitude of the tone from increasing to decreasing under control of the subject. The subject is instructed to press a hand-held button whenever and as long as he hears the tone. The tone grows at a constant rate, in dB per second, as long as the button is not pressed and decays at the same rate during the time the button is pressed. The resulting tracing when the patient follows this procedure to keep the tone just audible looks like the solid jagged line in Fig. 69. Ignoring the interweaving broken line for the moment, we can see that this patient began to hear the tone when it was at about a

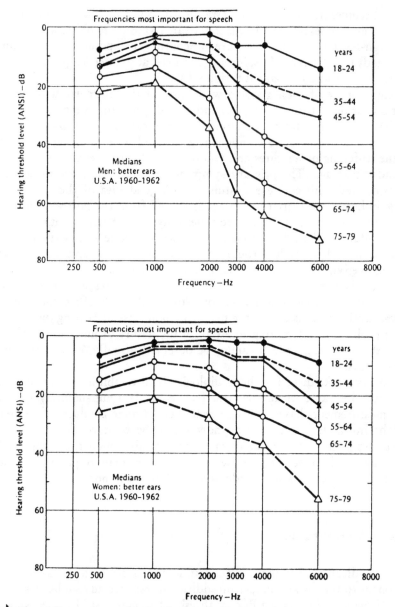

Fig. 68. The median pure tone hearing loss for both men and women as a function of age. These values are for the better ear for the individuals measured. (From U.S. Public Health Service Publication, No. 1000, Series 11, No. 11)

32 dB Hearing Level at about 100 Hz, since this is when the push of the button made the tone start to decrease. At about 24 dB HL the tone had disappeared and the release of the button caused it to begin to grow again, etc.

If the test is repeated with the tone pulsing every 400 milliseconds (200 msec on—200 msec off), the tracing for a patient with a conductive loss will simply interweave with the continuous tracing, as in Fig. 69. A similar pair

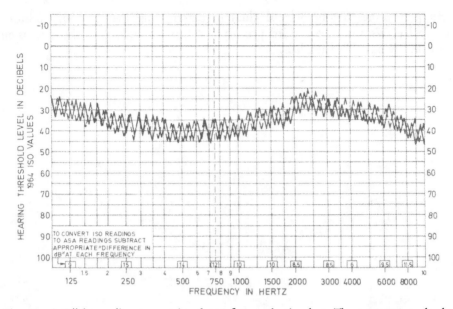

Fig. 69. A Békésy audiometer tracing for a flat conductive loss. The tone sweeps slowly over the frequency range as the listener keeps it moving above and below audibility.
(See text)

of tracings will result from testing a normal-hearing subject, except that both tracings will lie much nearer the 0 dB HL line.

The usefulness of the Békésy audiogram emerges, however, when the loss is not a conductive loss. If instead of the tracings for the continuous tone and the pulsed tone interweaving, the double trace looks like Fig. 70, the probability is quite high that the trouble is in the cochlea. Notice that at about 1 kHz the threshold for pulsed tones begins to be better than for the continuous tone. Although the tracings run parallel through the high frequency range, the threshold for pulsed tones is about 20 dB better than for the uninterrupted tone. But we might note also that once the separation has begun the tracing for the continuous tone looks quite different than before. Whereas in the frequency range where the tracings overlapped it appears to take the patient a goodly fraction of a second to decide that the tone was audible or inaudible, it now seems to move above and below threshold much more positively.

A closer look at this increased definiteness of thresholds is afforded by taking the same kind of tracing pair at a single frequency rather than having the frequency continually changing. This can be seen in Fig. 71, where it is again evident that the tracing for the continuous tone reaches an asymptote and stays parallel with the upper trace. These tracings that maintain a fixed separation and show narrowed swings on separating are known as Type II tracings. The overlapping pair shown in Fig. 68 is called Type I. The situation is not really quite so clear-cut as these examples make it seem. Many variations on these curves come from measurements in the clinic, and these should be considered simply the prototypes. It does require some considerable expertise to differentiate types validly in individual cases. Nevertheless, Békésy audiometry furnishes highly helpful clues in determining the locus of auditory difficulty. We shall see a third prototype when we move into the discussion of neurally based hearing loss.

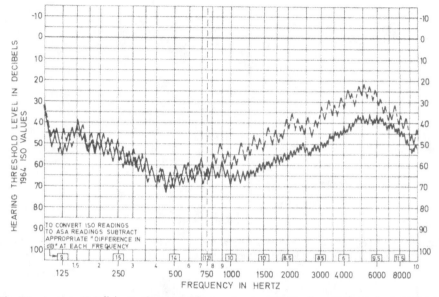

Fig. 70. A type II Békésy audiogram. The continuous tracing drops below the pulsed-tone tracing (broken line) at about 1 kHz, but separates by no more than 20 dB as the two tracings continue. The beginning of narrow swings in the continuous-tone tracing coincides with the separation of the two tracings

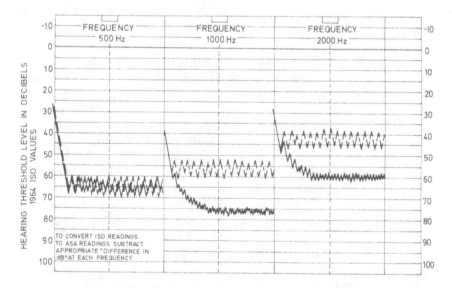

Fig. 71. A fixed-frequency Békésy audiogram showing the relation between pulsed- and continuous-tone tracings expected from a patient who gives a Type II swept-frequency tracing. Separation remains about the same once it reaches asymptote and the narrowed swing occurs only at those frequencies where the tracings separate

Other Cochlear Tests

There are also additional indices of difficulty in the cochlea. They are not easy to corroborate, since the whole process is a somewhat circular one in the following sense. Initially, an entire battery of tests and symptoms is used to arrive at a diagnosis of inner ear involvement. Then, in an effort to simplify the identification of locus, frequently specific tests are applied to these same cases to ascertain whether for future cases the simpler single measure can supplant the more elaborate set of tests and history.

In this fashion an abnormally rapid growth of loudness has been associated statistically with trouble in the inner ear. The clearest demonstration results from testing cases of unilateral inner-ear involvement. Shown in Fig. 72 is the result of a test called the Alternate Binaural Loudness Balance (ABLB) test. Tones of about $1/2$ second duration with smooth onset and decay are presented alternately to the two ears. The patient is instructed either to make the signals in the two ears equally loud or to indicate to the experimenter when they are equally loud, depending on who controls the level of the tone.

If we plotted the result of such a procedure for a pair of normal ears, the plotted points—indicating the levels where the two tones were matched in loudness—would lie on or close to the dotted diagonal line. If we made a similar measurement on a patient with an equal conductive loss in both ears, the points would still lie near the diagonal, but there would be no points near the lower left corner of the plot since neither ear hears low-level tones. If the patient had a 40 dB conductive loss, but only in one ear, then the points would fall on or near the dashed line—parallel to the diagonal.

The interesting case is portrayed by the solid line. It can be seen from the first point plotted that this patient has a much greater loss in one ear than the other at the frequency tested. When the tone is just above threshold in the poorer ear (50 dB HL), it requires a tone just above threshold in the better ear to match it in loudness. But if the worse-ear tone is raised just another 5 dB, it

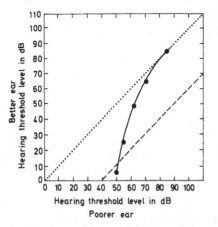

Fig. 72. A plot for showing the form of binaural loudness balance. The better ear is used as a standard for testing rate of loudness growth in the poorer ear. Amount of loudness recruitment may be regarded as the slope of the line

requires an increase of 15 dB in the better ear to match it in loudness. Apparently loudness grows much more rapidly, for a given decibel change, in the bad ear than in the good ear. This more rapid growth of loudness has been called recruitment in clinical audiology. Whether it is related to the general phenomenon of neural recruitment well known in neurophysiology has not been well established. It does seem to occur in this extreme form only in ears which by other indices have difficulties of cochlear origin.

The unusually rapid growth of loudness and the comparative suddenness of movement above and below auditory threshold at some frequencies, as shown in the Békésy tracings of Fig. 70 have led to the feeling that these patients can perceive smaller changes in intensity than other listeners, particularly at low levels. If this were measurably true, it would add another test for cochlear site of involvement. Such an additional test would be welcome, since, as we have indicated, Békésy tracings do not always take the easily interpretable form of Fig. 70, and there is seldom enough sensitivity difference between ears to make the Alternate Binaural Loudness Balance test conclusive.

In the terms of our previous discussion of the psychoacoustics of the ear, the prediction would be that these patients have a smaller just noticeable difference in intensity than normal. A number of tests of this just noticeable difference have been tried in audiology clinics, but the one now in most common use—especially in America—is the Short Increment Sensitivity Index (SISI) test. The procedure for this test is best understood by referring to Fig. 73. A steady tone 20 dB above the patient's threshold is presented at the test frequency and every 5 seconds its amplitude changes smoothly to a higher value as shown. The amplitude rise takes place over 50 msec, so there is very little energy scattered to other frequencies. The amplitude rise is equivalent to a 1 dB increase ($\approx 11\,\%$). This is not enough to be heard by the normal listener at these low signal levels (see p. 72). But the listener with cochlear involvement is very apt to hear these small increments at high frequencies.

Whether a common factor underlies the rapid growth of loudness, the abrupt entry of the tone above threshold and the increased sensitivity to small changes in amplitude is still a matter for conjecture. They do not occur consistently in all patients, but any one of them occurs more frequently in

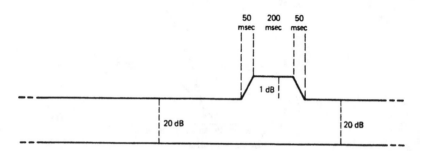

Fig. 73. The time sequence for a single trial of the Short Increment Sensitivity Index (SISI) test. For the standard test, the increment shown occurs once every 5 seconds. The patient can be given practice trials on increments larger than 1 dB. During the formal test, blank trials should be inserted

patients who, by other signs, have troubles of cochlear origin. Consequently, the Short Increment Sensitivity Index, the narrowed Békésy tracing and, where testable, the abnormally rapid growth of loudness in the poorer ear are all used as partial, but not conclusive, indications of trouble in the cochlea.

Abnormally rapid growth of loudness—now commonly called recruitment—appears to be a fairly reliable sign of cochlear involvement. Thus it is fortunate that another measure of this behavior is available that does not depend on the difference between the two ears of the same patient. The reasoning is as follows: The acoustic reflex appears to be triggered by the loudness response. In cases where no abnormal loudness growth is present, the level adequate to trigger the reflex should be Hearing Loss (dB) + Normal Reflex Level. For example, for the bad ear of the patient measured for Fig. 72, with a threshold at 55 dB HL and an expected tonal reflex threshold of 85 dB Sensation Level, one would not expect to elicit a reflex in that ear until the level exceeded the 110 dB HL limit of most audiometers. However, if by 85 dB HL in the bad ear, the tone is as loud as it would be in the normal ear—as in the case portrayed in Fig. 72—, and if the reflex *is* loudness mediated, then ears with abnormal loudness growth will show reflex activation at lower-than-expected sensation levels. The advantage of this measure over some other indices of inner ear dysfunction is that it is taken with the tympanometric device discussed earlier and requires no voluntary response from the patient. This can be very useful for testing young children (Jerger *et al.*, 1974), or on occasion others for whom response is difficult.

From our discussion thus far of inner-ear loss, it appears that nothing is amiss except for a loss of sensitivity. It is not obvious that any devastating effects would accrue to an abnormal rate of loudness growth or an increased sensitivity to small amplitude increments. But many of these patients, even before they appear at the audiology clinic or the doctor's office are aware that simply making sound louder does not completely solve the problem. The difficulty is most noticeable, of course, when listening to speech; and the reaction of such a patient is apt to be "Yes, it's loud enough, but not *clear* enough to understand".

The extent of loss of speech communication is ultimately the practical measure of the severity of a hearing loss. Tests of hearing for speech have always been used for estimating the degree of loss, but have become sufficiently quantifiable only with the advent of electronic reproducing equipment. How nearly speech perception measured in the audiology clinic mirrors degree of difficulty in everyday reception of speech is still debatable, but much effort has been expended in standardizing the testing of hearing for speech. As a result, two major types of speech testing are part of the audiologic test battery. The first, and simplest, of these is testing for speech thresholds. One form of this is the Speech Detection Threshold (SDT) usually measured by exposing the patient to continuous recorded discourse and noting at what level on the Hearing Level dial the patient can just detect that the speech signal is present.

In order for this measure to be comparable from one clinic and one test to another some agreement must be reached about the level of speech at 0 dB Hearing Level. This will necessarily be arbitrary, since the different sounds of speech (the phonemes, if one wishes to break it down to that degree) vary in level as much as 28—30 dB from the strong [ɔ] sound to the weak [θ] (unvoiced th). The method of specifying the level in speech test material is to record on the test tape a calibration tone at 1 kHz that drives the VU meter to the same level that the meter reaches during peak energies of the spoken test words. For audiometer calibration purposes, the sound pressure level that this calibration tone produces in the standard 6 cc coupler is called the sound pressure level of that recorded speech sample.

Since the salient purpose of speech testing is to test understanding rather than awareness, a much more useful measure than Speech Detection Threshold is the Speech Reception Threshold. This refers to the setting of the Hearing Level dial required for the patient to repeat one half the presented test words correctly. The test words in this case are a restricted set of Spondee (bi-syllabic, equal stress) words such as pancake, stairwell, cowboy, etc. They have the useful property of being equally intelligible, and they therefore make a relatively homogeneous set of test items. The speech transmission channel of a calibrated audiometer is set so that for a normal listener, on the average, one half of these words will be correctly repeated when the Hearing Level dial is at zero. Since the major clues for these words are likely the tones of the vowel formants, we might predict a constant relation between the SRT and the pure tone threshold in the frequencies where the sensation levels of speech are highest, i.e., where speech first comes above threshold. The audiometric frequencies 500, 1000 and 2000 are often referred to by audiologists as the speech frequencies, and the average Hearing Level for pure tone testing at these frequencies is compared to the Hearing Level for SRT as a quick check on the consistency of testing.

Over a large sample with different shapes of audiograms, the correlation between the average HL of the three frequencies and the HL for Spondee threshold was very high for the group with flat audiograms ($r=0.97$) Carhart and Porter, 1971). Even for groups with irregular pure-tone audiograms, the correlation dropped very little, the lowest coefficient being close to 0.90. The mean HL's for the Spondee threshold and the three-frequency tone average were also surprisingly close, differing by only about 1 dB for the group with flat audiograms. This has to be considered essentially fortuitous, since there is no inherent reason that the threshold as set by the VU meter reading for peaks of speech sounds should agree that closely with the average threshold for the middle frequencies. It is primarily empirical assurance that the Spondee SRT as a cross check on the pure-tone audiogram is quite useful. It is not always that simple, since for individual patients with abrupt discontinuities in the audiogram, the average of the pure tone threshold may be a comparatively poor index of the level needed to understand half the Spondee words.

With some caution, then, the SRT is used in two ways in the audiology clinic: (1) It is employed as the estimated zero sensation level for speech tests, and (2) it is used as a rough cross check on pure tone testing.

Most of us, on some occasion, experience speech that is sufficiently loud, but still not intelligible. It may be a bad radio or telephone transmission, which, even though noise free in the masking sense, sounds garbled and is very difficult to follow. This may happen also if our informant has a very bad "accent" that keeps us from following what is being said, even though he may (misguidedly) speak much more loudly in an effort to be understood. There is, in other words, a common-sense impression that the understanding of a speech message depends on a factor or factors other than the raising of its threshold by interfering noise. It is well established empirically that patients with non-conductive losses fail to repeat some proportion of test words correctly even when the level has been raised 30—40 dB above their speech threshold. This auditory behavior, for reasons that are not worth tracing, has come to be labeled poor speech discrimination; and the measurement of this above-threshold component of speech perception in the audiology clinic is called speech discrimination testing.

The most common form of Word Discrimination Test (WDT) is a standard list of monosyllabic words. One presumed use of such a test is as a measure of communication difficulty. At this point, though, we are concerned with cochlear disorders, and the question is whether such a list of words can be used to aid in the diagnosis of the *kind* of loss presented by the patient. It would be convenient also if certain kinds of errors in recognizing the words of speech tests were made by listeners with one kind of loss, but not by those with losses of different origin.

The test list is presented according to a standard format, with some variation from clinic to clinic. Usually the baseline for setting the level of presentation of the words is the SRT, meaning the setting of the Hearing Level dial at which the patient repeated correctly 50 % of the Spondee words presented. The chosen list of words for the Speech Discrimination Test is presented at a dial setting 30 dB above SRT in some clinics, 40 dB above in some others, and sometimes at a separately determined "comfort level for speech". This flexibility can be defended on the grounds that for this kind of speech testing, level is not critical once we are 30 dB above the SRT. Somewhat opposed to that point of view is the idea that information about the kind of loss can be garnered from testing at several levels and plotting level of presentation *vs* percent of words correct.

Such plots are, in fact, quite informative about the behavior of different kinds of item for speech testing. Obviously at a sufficiently low level none of the words will be understood. As the level is raised past the point where a few items are heard correctly, an increasingly greater proportion can be reported correctly. Both the starting level and the rate at which the proportion correct grows differ for different kinds of speech sample. Some of the rationale for selecting tests currently in use has come from such plots, as portrayed in Fig. 74. We have already spoken of the relative steepness of the curve for Spondee words and the resulting efficiency for estimating speech threshold.

The test most widely used at levels above threshold are monosyllabic word tests. The two rightmost curves illustrate the point that if speech is perceived as disorted it may not become completely intelligible no matter how high the level. The material for the curve marked "Hughes recording" is only slightly "distorted" by virtue of being rapidly and carelessly articulated.

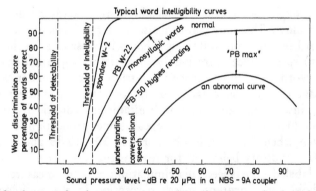

Fig. 74. Idealized curves for the increase in word intelligibility as level of the speech signal is increased. Sound Pressure Level of speech is a rapidly varying quantity, but a standard for speech audiometry has been the Sound Pressure Level of a 1 kHz tone that drives the VU meter on the speech audiometer to the same level as the peaks of speech. For monosyllabic test words, a carrier (introductory) phrase is usually used and the SPL is defined relative to the carrier peak, with the words spoken with equal vocal effort. An intelligibility curve for sentences would look almost like the one for the Spondee words. These should be regarded only as typical curves. Considerable variation comes with different talkers and different word lists. (From Davis and Silverman, 1978)

Actually it might be argued that it is the only *undistorted* sample by the yardstick of everyday pronunciation! Materials for the other curves undoubtedly err on the side of overarticulation compared to everyday speech.

The curve labeled abnormal represents one type of plot from testing a patient with a non-conductive loss. Whether this type of "roll-over" in the curve occurs to a significant degree with losses of cochlear origin is a matter of some disagreement (Jerger and Jerger, 1971). The occurrence of marked roll-over as level increases may be indicative of a neural loss. If further data establish that this difference in shape of speech intelligibility curve can help substantially in separating the two kinds of loss, then measuring speech discrimination at a single level above SRT, as many clinics now do, may turn out to be an unwise shortcut.

In testing a given patient, what must be weighed against the possible efficacy of such complete performance curves as those shown in Fig. 74 is the difficulty of making a more elaborate measurement and including enough items at each level to assure reasonable reliability. Currently most clinics still opt for a single Speech Discrimination score, obtained by presenting the test words at a level comfortably above the patient's SRT. Even this performance by the patient could conceivably be diagnostically useful. There have been several attempts to ascertain whether certain types of errors in speech sound identification are empirically associated with certain types of hearing loss. This might occur because certain spectral regions are more important in some sounds than others, or it might mean the perception of rapidly-changing time patterns is crucial to the processing of some sounds more than others. Attempts to associate kinds of speech discrimination errors with type of hearing loss have not been successful enough to have much influence on speech discrimination testing in the clinic.

VIIIth Nerve Problems 14

There is some evidence, however, that even though the pattern of speech-sound confusion may not be useful in indicating the kind of loss, separation of cochlear from VIIIth nerve loss may be possible by plotting the kind of performance curves shown in Fig. 74. Jerger and Jerger (1971) ran such curves on a number of patients, using phonetically balanced (PB) monosyllabic words. These patients had hearing loss diagnosed either as cochlear or VIIIth nerve. Patients with cochlear disorders did not usually show the "roll-over" of the curve as suggested in the figure. Instead they reached a plateau and stayed at that level, usually at some percentage of correct responses well below 100. Patients with VIIIth nerve involvement, by contrast, performed more nearly as the "abnormal" curve implies. They reached a maximum at some level well above threshold, but then as the level was further increased they were able to identify a smaller and smaller proportion of the words.

Just as we saw with the problem of separating conductive from non-conductive losses, the separation of cochlear and neural losses cannot be accomplished with a single test. Some patients with cochlear losses also show the roll-over phenomenon, though it occurs with greater relative frequency in neural losses.

Further confidence in placing the site of the disorder can come from the results of the Tone Decay Test (TDT). It works in the following manner. If a normal hearer is given a sustained tone at a level 5 dB above his threshold, he will continue to hear the tone as long as he attends carefully and remains quiet. For persons with neurally based losses, however, the tone will fade away in 10 to 15 seconds. If at that point the signal is increased by 5 dB, the tone is heard again, and again remains audible for only about 10—15 seconds. For some patients, this may continue to happen through 5 or 6 such increments.

In the most frequently used form, the tester continues to raise the tone in 5 dB steps until it remains audible for at least 60 seconds. The amount by which the tone has been raised above its original threshold when this Tone Decay Test, since the continuous tracing gives the impression the patient 60-second duration is achieved is reported as the amount of tone decay. If this amounts to 30 dB the test may not be pursued further, since this is considered sufficient to indicate marked tone decay.

Again we do not have a test that by itself can cleanly separate cochlear involvement from neural. Owens (1964) demonstrated that patients with Meniere's disease, a cochlear involvement, also show tone decay, although if one traces the time course of the disappearance of the tone for each 5 dB increase the pattern is different for cochlear and neural cases. In practice, the Tone Decay Test is used as part of a battery for ascertaining which is the site of difficulty.

In addition to speech test results and the Tone Decay Test, the comparison of pulsed and continuous Békésy tracings can give a clue to the nature of the hearing loss. The tracing can be a rather distinctive one as in the example of Fig. 75. It may be testing virtually the identical elements tested by the Tone Decay Test, since the continuous tracing gives the impression the patient is tracking the result of tone decay at threshold. It is also useful to know how the traced pattern looks when stimulating a given cochlear segment continually, rather than moving on as in the conventional Békésy pattern. Such fixed-frequency tracings might have the look of those in Fig. 76, indicating that the sound is kept close to threshold even though it grows fairly rapidly in intensity. Frequently what the patient hears is not tonal, but has the character of a hissing or frying sound. Occasionally very similar tracings can come from patients with cochlear involvement—particularly those with sudden hearing loss, so again the test battery approach is preferable to the single test.

Acoustic reflexes can also be of some help in making this distinction between cochlear and VIIIth nerve involvement. Once other measures have

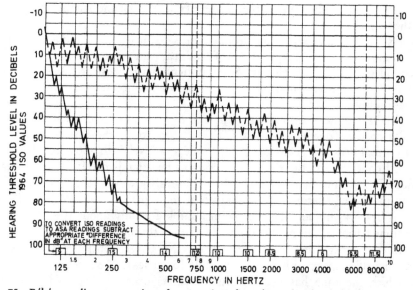

Fig. 75. Békésy audiometer tracings for a patient for whom the threshold for continuous tones shifts extremely rapidly. This is labeled a Type III audiogram, and along with other tests can be helpful in identifying VIIIth nerve involvement

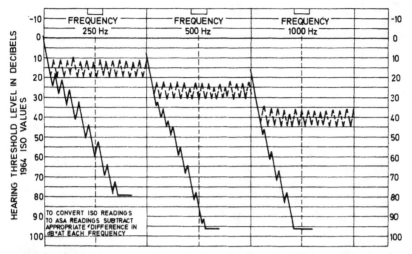

Fig. 76. Békésy fixed-frequency tracings showing the dramatic difference between threshold for a pulsed tone (solid line) and for a continous tone for a Type III audiogram. For the continous tone, the patient's threshold shift is nearly as rapid as the increase in level of the automatic audiometer, so the tone never gets far above threshold, even out to the audiometer limits

established the fact that the loss is non-conductive, the level at which the reflex can be elicited is a useful index of site of lesion. Usually, if the reflex appears at or close to the usual SPL in spite of a loss of sensitivity, then recruitment must be present and the cochlea is involved. Occasionally even with a neural loss reflexes may appear at a lower level than the amount of loss would lead one to predict. In this case the muscle action is not sustained. It adapts quickly, and some clinics have been measuring this course of reflex decay to help in the cochlear *vs* neural decision. The implication seems to be that when the dysfunction is cochlear, recruitment in the form of near-normal loudnesss-intensity relations above threshold is to be expected, and that therefore the reflex threshold for the middle ear muscles will not be shifted. A further implication with some types of neural loss is that where scattered sporadic nerve fiber loss is the rule, the reflex threshold for any given frequency will not be shifted. But where a spatially concentrated loss of fiber function has occurred—as with pressure from a tumor—certain frequencies will show a shift in threshold or a reflex decay with continued stimulation. For cases where the loss itself is so severe that reflexes are simply out of reach of audiometer levels, the decision about cochlear or neural site of involvement may be only academic.

For less severe losses and particularly for younger persons, the distinction between cochlear and neural loss may be an important one. If VIIIth nerve type of loss indicates pressure on the nerve or the lower brain stem from a tumor, a different regimen of monitoring and diagnosis is indicated than would be the case for a cochlear involvement. The point is that the audiologist can be of considerable help to the neuro-otologist or otologist if the indications for neural involvement can be cleanly separated from those pointing toward cochlear dysfunction.

15 Threshold Shift

We saw, in our discussion of the ear's response to any tone, that there ensued a short period after stimulation during which the sensitivity had not returned completely to normal. For stronger tones this period of reduced sensitivity is even longer. Thus our concern focuses on whether this failure to return quickly to normal sensitivity indicates an increasing danger that with enough stimulation some permanent impairment will result.

Even without laboratory testing we have known for a long time that ears exposed to unusually high level sounds for long periods show permanent loss of sensitivity. But since many of our activities involve being immersed in a sound field of medium level for relatively long periods we need to know more about the upper limits of safe levels for exposure to sound. If one habitually spends long hours close to the seemingly innocuous hum of the refrigerator or an exhaust fan, will some noticeable hearing impairment result? Can the musician or the addicted hi-fi listener be confident that as average preferred levels of music seem to rise his hearing will remain suitably sensitive to softer sounds?

There is some reassurance regarding the effects of medium-level, medium duration sounds from the work of Hirsh and Bilger (1955). For exposures to tones (1 kHz) at levels between 20 and 80 dB above threshold and for durations up to 4 minutes, temporary threshold shifts (TTS) of only a few dB are the rule. From much other evidence we know that long-term effects from such levels and durations are small enough to be within the range of the normal variation of auditory threshold. It is a matter of great interest in the study of the operation of the auditory system that such a loss of normal sensitivity persists for seconds after exposure to even low-level sounds, but it certainly is not an immediate danger signal. Because it appears that the system requires some "silent" time to recover completely from almost any stimulation, early workers referred to the phenomenon as auditory fatigue. The more operational term, which we will use throughout, is Temporary Threshold Shift.

The course of recovery for these medium-level, medium-duration signals —noise as well as tones—is relatively smooth and reasonably rapid, being complete within a few minutes. To what extent it is a continuation of the residual or forward masking process is not easy to determine. It may well be a combination of the effects of relative refractory periods of the nerves and natural replenishment of necessary metabolic material. Undoubtedly it has its effect on the hearing of suddenly softer sounds following an intense sound, such as special orchestral effects or weak sounds of speech immediately following strong sounds, and in that sense is seen to be an extension of forward masking.

Recovery from stronger sounds of greater duration presents a different picture. Sounds reaching levels around 80 to 100 dB SPL or greater leave the auditory system in a state of less-than-normal sensitivity for a longer period. Furthermore the sequence of recovery as portrayed in Fig. 77 is more complex, as though possibly several factors may be contributing. At these levels, concern over the likelihood of cumulative effects that mean less than complete recovery is very real. The problem is to ascertain whether this is so without risking loss to the ears being tested. One possibility is to conduct the test on animals, but testing threshold and threshold changes in animals is difficult at best and has been possible only in behavioral studies. We do not as yet have reliable electrical or chemical measures of very small sensitivity changes.

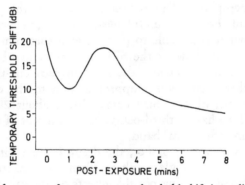

Fig. 77. The course of recovery from temporary threshold shift immediately after exposure. This is an average of many experimental measures. Why the partial relapse after recovery has begun has never been fully understood. (Modified from Hirsh and Bilger, 1955)

One way to study the relation between TTS and the onset of Permanent Threshold Shift (PTS) is to measure, whenever the opportunity arises, the onset and progression of loss in those workers who *are* involved in working situations that necessitate exposure to levels suspected to be high enough to lead to eventual hearing loss. A great many such measurements have been made, under as nearly controlled conditions as practically possible. As a consequence we do have at least interim answers to questions about maximum safe levels of exposure.

A great many questions still persist in arriving at such empirically-derived estimates. Is the Noise Induced Hearing Loss (NIHL) additive with other contributors to hearing loss? One such contributor, as we measure workers over a period of years, is the average loss with advancing age. This comes about from so many different causes that the usual procedure, in estimating the effect of a given exposure, is to correct a measured NIHL for the age of the worker. In addition to the average loss attributable, from statistical considerations, to age itself, some damage to hearing may have resulted from other incidental high-level exposures, from unusual exposure to certain medicinal drugs or from other physiologic insults. Whenever we do need to know, perhaps also for workmen's compensation purposes, how much hearing loss is attributable to industrial noise exposure in a given case, we really ought to have a pre-employment audiogram, because any individual's history is apt to be affected significantly by these other contributors to loss. But only in a few fortunate instances will we have such pre-exposure baseline information. Lacking such information in using already-exposed workers for arriving at a reasonable estimate of safe levels we can take the next best step of measuring, where possible, representative samples and correcting for estimated average amounts of loss attributable to other factors. We saw a portrayal of expected loss in the general population for different ages in Fig. 68 (p. 136).

The first step in determining safe levels from exposure history is to measure the level of the noise. The Sound Level meter, as its name implies, is a device specifically designed to measure the Sound Pressure Level at the location of its microphone. This is usually placed at the position of the listener's ear or head. For more useful measurement the meter may include a set of filters so that it is possible to plot a rough spectrum of the noise. This may take the form of showing the SPL in each octave band or possibly a finer subdivision of the spectrum, the level in each one-third octave band. This latter is rather a convenient approximation to the critical bandwidth of the ear, the width of one-third octave being about 26 % of the center frequency. Thus if we have a third-octave spectrum plot of the noise we know roughly the level in each critical band.

Usually, however, wisely or not, the desire is for a simpler specification of the noise, preferably a single number. When the measurement is made for the express purpose of assessing possible effects on the ear, a special equalization curve is used in measuring the overall level. Employing this equalization gives the meter a frequency response roughly resembling the transmission characteristic of the ear. We saw the shape of this curve and some of its contributing components early in our discussion of the ear (Fig. 3). This setting is known as the "A" scale of the Sound Level meter, and when this curve has been used in the measurement of sound pressure levels, the result is designated as dBA. Levels for some typical sounds are shown in Table 2.

It is apparent, even from this partial list, that most of us on occasion have our ears exposed to sounds that approach or exceed 90—100 dBA. How much of such exposure can occur without having some lasting effect on our hearing? We have seen that no very simple answer comes from exploring within the range where it is safe to produce temporary threshold shift, and so we measure samples of workers already exposed to different levels for different durations. Still the answer is not easily given. For one thing, as seen in Fig. 78, it depends on what frequency range we consider important. This result,

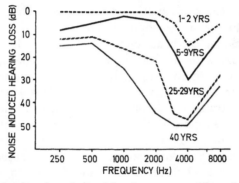

Fig. 78. Area of hearing loss from industrial noise exposure. The noise was strongest in the frequency range from 500 to 2000 Hz. In most such losses the pure tone loss is not a full indication of the degree of communication handicap. (From Taylor *et al.*, 1965)

Table 2. *Some typical noises and their dBA levels*

Overall Level (dBA)		Community or Outdoor	Home or Indoor
120	Uncomfortably loud	Chain saw (operator), 110 dBA	Rock 'n' roll band, 108 to 114 dBA
		Jet flyover (1000 ft), 103 dBA	Symphony orchestra, 110 dBA
100	Very loud	Power mower, 96 dBA	
90		Motorcycles (25 ft), 90 dBA	
		Propeller aircraft flyover, (1000 ft) 88 dBA	Food blender, 88 dBA
		Diesel truck, 40 mph (50 ft) 84 dBA	
80	Moderately loud	Passenger car, 65 mph (25 ft) 77 dBA	Garbage disposal, 80 dBA Clothes washer, 78 dBA Living room music, 76 dBA Dishwasher, 75 dBA Television, 70 dBA
		Auto traffic, (near freeway) 64 dBA	Conversation, 65 dBA
		Air conditioning unit (20 ft), 60 dBA	
50	Quiet	Light traffic (100 ft), 50 dBA	

from a particular sample of workers exposed to noise that was strongest in the range from 500 to 2000 Hz, is typical of what happens with many noises that have energy spread throughout the spectrum. Losses in the range 3000 to 5000 Hz occur earliest even though the spectral maximum of the exposure noise may be considerably lower. A little later in our discussion we shall see that a similar result accrues from explosive sound wave episodes—the major damage occurs in this 3000—5000 Hz range. We saw earlier that this is the resonance region of the mechanical auditory system. Békésy's calculation of the amplitude of the basilar membrane in human cadaver preparations driven at high amplitudes indicates an increase in amplitude of 10 : 1 between 1500 Hz and 3 kHz, with the sound pressure held constant (Békésy, 1960, p. 173). Whether this accounts completely for the phenomenon is debatable.

Much of the past measurement of hearing loss from industrial noise exposure has concentrated on the loss at frequencies in the range of 500 to 2000 Hz, since this is supposedly the frequency range important to the understanding of speech. In an effort to get a manageable view of the effect of frequency, level and duration of exposure on the eventual loss, we can take the average hearing loss at 500 Hz, 1 kHz and 2 kHz to indicate the most important segment of the hearing loss, take a population with long exposure and select subsamples within that exposed population that have worked in different levels of the noise. The results for one such study are shown in Fig. 79. These measurements are on people who had worked for forty years in the noise level shown on the abscissa. Their losses are averaged over the three frequencies and corrected for the average (non-exposed) population loss at their age.

At least two important points follow from this idealized graph. The first is that not all the persons exposed at 95 dBA show the same average amount of loss. This could be shown more dramatically if we plotted the same data for higher levels of exposure where total losses are greater. Such considerations have generated the notion that some ears are more susceptible to loss from noise exposure than others—that there are "tender" and "tough" ears. Efforts to verify this from measurements of Temporary Threshold Shift and correlations with other indices within the exposed population have not identified any useful physiological parallels.

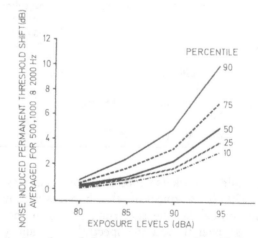

Fig. 79. The distribution of speech-frequency pure tone loss. These are workers who have been working for forty years at the exposure level shown. Amount of loss has been corrected for the average loss of non-exposed persons of the same age. These levels are considered to encompass the range between safe and unsafe exposure. (From Johnson, 1973)

The second point is that at 90 dBA there is a change in the rate of loss increase with increasing level of exposure. From a great many other such measurements and from corroborating data from animal experiments the "safe" level for an 8-hr working day exposure is taken to be 90 dBA. One simple rule about other durations asserts that for every halving of the duration one can add 3 dB to the safe level, for example, for an exposure of 4 hrs 93 dBA could be tolerated, for 2 hrs 96 dBA, etc.

It should be remembered that applying this rule of thumb amounts to the grossest oversimplification. Damage Risk Criteria evolved by a group of experts for the Committee on Hearing, Bioacoustics and Biomechanics of the National Academy of Sciences take the form of 11 graphs relating frequency, duration and temporal characteristics of the exposure sounds. Anyone involved with the assessment of a specific noise should dig much deeper into recommendations for safe levels than our interest has taken us here.

What we have considered so far is noise that is relatively unchanging in time. Quite different considerations apply to sounds of an explosive nature. Gunshots may be the most familiar example. Fig. 80 shows the instantaneous sound pressure from a pistol shot. The peak pressure reached is extremely high, but because it occurs over such a short period the usual meter would greatly underestimate the level. To a lesser degree this is also true of other impulse sounds, such as air hammers or helicopters. In extreme cases, these can cause damage to the ear at levels that do not show a very high reading on the meter simply because the meter is much slower than the mechanical part of the ear.

Pressure waves of this type, when they exceed about 130—140 dB can cause structural damage to the ear. Experiments with animals have shown that in such instances clumps of hair cells may be torn loose from the supporting membrane. The area of maximum damage is still the 3000—5000 Hz segment. Paradoxically, in those instances in which the tympanic membrane ruptures from the pressure the outcome is more fortunate since, even though the episode is more painful, the inner ear is apt to be undamaged. Perforations in the eardrum will heal or can be repaired, but very little recovery takes place after this type of damage to the inner ear.

There are a number of things to be considered about the hearing loss following long-term noise exposure. Since the loss incurred is not a conductive loss, essentially the same mechanical events are occurring as long as the person continues to suffer the same exposure. Evidence indicates that hearing damage will continue to occur until some asymptote is reached, determined by the nature and level of the noise. Persons who discover losses still in the early stage do well to curtail the exposure, either by changing location or by wearing suitable ear protection.

The pattern of discovery of early loss from noise exposure is an interesting and predictable one. In the days of mechanical wrist watches, it might happen that the first indication was an inability to detect the ticking of the watch when trying to make certain it was running. Usually, however, the discovery comes later when the person notes that things are a little more difficult to hear in the evening than in the morning. If nothing is done at that point and the loss progresses it may reach a point where hearing is noticeably better on

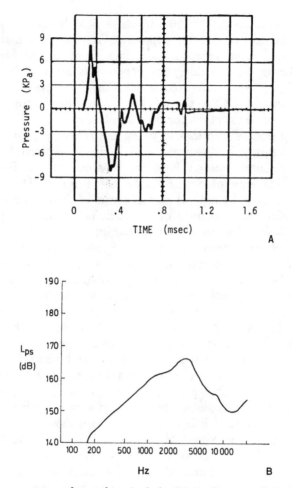

Fig. 80. Sound pressure waveform of a pistol shot. At a distance of about 0.5 meter this reaches a peak equivalent Sound Pressure Level of 169 dB. This large pressure excursion lasts for only 10's of microseconds in this instance. The spectrum is broad with a peak around 3 kHz. Exposure to repeated waves of this sort will definitely lead to a troublesome hearing loss

the weekend than other days. Finally, if preventive measures still have not been taken, only vacation times bring noticeably better hearing. How far the loss progresses with continued exposure depends, as indicated above, on the level and nature of the noise.

The progression described is just what we might expect from our knowledge of the behavior of temporary threshold shifts. At what point irreversible damage actually begins is not known, since some evidence indicates that "thresholds" will still measure the same even when a number of hair cell or neural units are missing. Keeping exposure within the established Damage Risk Criterion is the only safe procedure—another instance where an ounce of prevention may be worth its weight in gold.

Evoked Response Audiometry 16

The last decade has brought a great increase in the use of electrophysiologic tests of auditory function. Such tests are possible because with modern technology evidence of the electrical activity of the system can be picked up with non-invasive, or nearly non-invasive, techniques. These tests are especially useful for children who cannot yet respond to the usual behavioral testing regimen. The importance of early assessment of hearing dysfunction can scarcely be overemphasized. Electric response tests, therefore, which in skillful hands can be reliable on infants of a few months age, can be extremely valuable in early assurance and guidance of parents, physicians and others concerned with the child's training.

The technique takes advantage of the fact that neural activity is electrical activity, and since the tissues of the head conduct electricity, the evidence of neural function is available at sites fairly well removed from the original electric generator. In addition, the method became practical with the availability of time-locked averaging devices as described below.

Cochleography

Of the techniques used, perhaps the easiest to envision is electrocochleography. This entails placing a pickup electrode fairly close to the cochlea and recording the electrical activity that the ear generates from an acoustic stimulus. The most direct technique used sends a recording needle through the tympanic membrane to contact the bony promontory that is the outer wall of the cochlea. This access can be seen in Fig. 81 where part of the tympanum has been cut away.

The voltage developed between this needle pickup electrode and a reference electrode on the earlobe is a relatively good indicator of electrical activity in the cochlea. Because the pickup points are close to the cochlea, fairly strong indica-

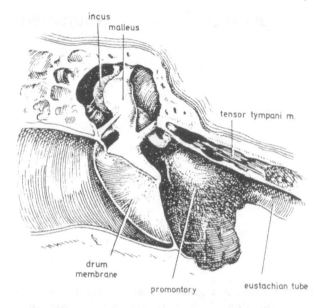

incus
malleus
tensor tympani m.
drum
membrane
promontory
eustachian tube

Fig. 81. Showing the path of access to the promontory where the cochlear microphonic
can be picked up by a needle through the tympanic membrane

tions of the neural action potential and the cochlear microphonic are available—of the order of 10 to 20 μv. Partly because tissue is a reasonable
conductor of electricity, other electric activity of the body is in evidence at
this same point, and must be regarded as noise that interferes with the cochlear
signal. Other electrical activity may in fact be at least as strong as the wanted
signal.

What makes it possible to isolate the desired activity is the technique of
signal-locked averaging. Each time a signal is delivered to the cochlea a
synchronizing pulse initiates an instant-to-instant recording of the activity
at the pickup electrode. Thus, for perhaps 10 msec following the onset of the
signal a number is recorded for the voltage at every 100 μsec interval. Voltages
for subsequent signals are averaged for each of these points on the synchronized
time line, and averaged, so that a composite average tracing is available after
n signals. Electrical activity not related to the signal presented is just as likely
to be negative as positive with respect to the reference point, so over many
trials unrelated activity will fail to sum coherently.

On the other hand, activity evoked by the signal will be relatively
consistent from one presentation to the next, and will yield a relatively noise-
free tracing of the electrical response(s) evoked by the signal. For instance, if
the unwanted activity is roughly the same amplitude as the evoked response,
it will be very difficult to ascertain the shape of the electrical response to the
stimulus. However, averaging 100 such responses by the technique just
described will yield a tracing with the amplitude of the signal about ten times
the amplitude of the averaged interference.

In recording electrical activity from the promontory another problem
arises. We recall from the discussion of electrical activity in the cochlea that

there are events other than the action potential that occur in synchrony with the acoustic signal. Of these, the cochlear microphonic is the most difficult to separate from the action potentials. Fortunately, in signal-locked averaging, these two can be fairly readily separated by taking advantage of the fact that the signal can be reversed in polarity on every other trial. Since the action potential does not change polarity, it will be reasonably well preserved in the averaging process as the microphonic, which follows the polarity of the signal, will average out. On the other hand, if the recording trace itself is reversed whenever the signal polarity is reversed, then the microphonic will be preserved and the action potential averaged out. Thus if one wishes, these two measures of cochlear activity can be assessed separately.

Vertex Electric Response

This procedure, as suggested, picks up the electrical activity of the cochlea fairly close to where it is generated. However, because of the necessity of piercing the eardrum, it does require that the patient be anesthetized and this is not pleasant and sometimes not practical for young patients. One attempt to overcome these objections makes use instead of an electrode in the external auditory canal. This also moves the pick-up point somewhat further from the source of the desired electric activity so that as much as 10 times as many signals may be necessary before the same averaged signal-to-noise is achieved. Quite fortuitously, because of the way electrical activity spreads through the head, a more practical pickup point is the vertex of the skull.

As we might guess, because this point is further from the ear, the level of the electrical activity from the ear is correspondingly lower. For a moderate-level signal, it is of the order of one microvolt or less. Consequently the ratio of wanted to unwanted electrical activity (the signal-to-noise ratio) is quite poor. By averaging 1000 or more click responses a reasonably stable record can be obtained, resembling that in Fig. 82.

One should remember that when the ear is stimulated by a sharp click nearly all segments of the basilar membrane will move, since a click contains energy over a wide range of frequency. Hence many cochlear neural units will respond electrically, and one might suppose that the electrical response would spread evenly over the approximately 5 msec that it takes the traveling wave from the click to traverse the length of the basilar membrane. A number of pertinent events occur that change such a prediction. The basal end of the basilar membrane, though it does respond best to very high frequencies drops off relatively slowly (≈ 12 dB/oct) in its response to lower frequencies. More than any other part of the membrane the basal segment tends to behave like a low pass filter with a broad pass band. This end of the membrane, then, will move nearly as a single segment in response to the click impulse. Thus synchronous neural discharges will come from this high-frequency end of the cochlea. The response is further modified by the resonance of the canal and the middle ear and the passband of the phone so that—at least at low signal

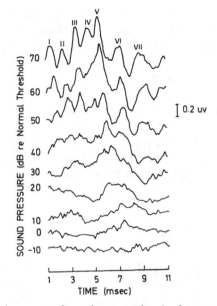

Fig. 82. Averaged electric response from the vertex for the first 11 msec following the signal. This represents the averaged response to 1024 clicks. When the clicks are at a 70 dB Sensation Level the separate peaks of the evoked response are very clearly identified. As the level drops, some peaks drop out; and by 20 dB above threshold the tracing is difficult to distinguish from noise. Wave V, however, remains identifiable longer than the others

levels—usually the portion contributing most heavily to the synchronous neural response out of the cochlea is the segment sensitive to about 2—4 kHz.

This form of the test, with repeated clicks and synchronous averaging of the signal recorded from the vertex electrode, is fairly simple to administer in the audiology clinic. It is frequently used for young children suspected of hearing loss who are too difficult or too young to test by behavioral methods. Sedation is usually used, but it does not require the presence of a physician.

One disadvantage of the test in this simplified form is that it does not test response at separate frequencies. Under good conditions, yielding a record like that in Fig. 82, the presence of the strongest peak (wave V) can be identified down to within 10—20 dB of behaviorally-measured threshold. Roughly speaking, these individual wave peaks that are discernible indicate the response of separate generators in the auditory brain stem. Wave I, which in practice is sometimes obscured by the presence of an electric artifact, is traceable to the activity of the VIIIth nerve; wave II is from the synchronous discharges of the cochlear nucleus; wave III from the superior olivary complex; wave IV probably from the lateral lemniscus, and wave V from the inferior colliculus.

Wave V not only persists as the level drops closer to threshold, but has another useful property in the behavior of its latency. Since these are all time-locked average tracings, the start of the trace bears a constant relation to the beginning of the acoustic signal. As the signal is attenuated by an additional 10 dB for successive tracings, wave V loses amplitude and also shows a systematic shift in its time relation to the acoustic signal onset. A reasonable conjecture is that as the level of signal drops, the response is more restricted to the region of greatest sensitivity, around 2—4 kHz, and the units of shortest latency—those closest to the basal end—no longer dominate the response.

This progression can be clinically useful as suggested in Fig. 83. Here is shown the latency of wave V as the click level is varied. If additional, short latency, units have progressively greater influence as the basilar excitation pattern spreads to the upper end, then it appears that a normal complement of high frequency fibers is functioning, and therefore hearing from about 2 kHz on up is normal. On similar reasoning, in an ear with recruitment, the latency *vs* level curve might be expected to show a steeper slope as additional units accrue more rapidly with increases in level. This is the case in Fig. 83 from Skinner and Glattke (1977).

Since one primary task of the cochlea is preliminary spectral analysis, it would be distinctly advantageous if Electric Response Audiometry could be made more specific to characteristic frequency segments of the cochlea—in other words, if something approaching a pure tone audiogram were the result. This should be possible with techniques currently in use (Davis, 1976), but to date (1980) there are few reports of its clinical use.

A small, and not insurmountable, problem arises because the spread of excitation on the basilar membrane is large even for a single frequency signal when that signal is well above threshold. Since the signal-locked averaging process favors synchronous activity, it might well be that the basal end of the membrane, where a large section moves in synchrony when it *does* respond to a middle or low frequency tone, contributes more heavily to the summed average than does the characteristic membrane segment for that frequency. This could be true even though the amplitude at the characteristic locus for

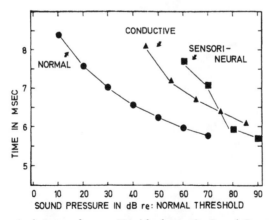

Fig. 83. The change in latency of wave V with change in Sound Pressure Level. As seen, there is gradually smaller delay between the click signal and the appearance of wave V in the response as level is increased. Theoretically the conductive loss curve should be just the same as the normal curve but moved to the right. But if the more rapid growth of loudness in recruitment means more nerve fibers active, the latency curve should drop more rapidly than normal—as it does. (From Skinner and Glattke, 1977)

the signal frequency is considerably greater than at the basal end. In any event, one cannot get a good estimate of the amount of loss at, say, the 500 Hz locus in the cochlea if other loci are contributing signal-synchronized neural bursts.

Yamada *et al.* (1978) shed a little light on the subject by measuring the evoked responses of patients with known hearing losses. They used short 500 Hz tone bursts as their repetitive signal. The electric response to such bursts is a 500 Hz "frequency following response" superimposed on the tracing of the slower electric responses. Their groups of patients were selected to have wide differences in the amount of low and high frequency loss. They noted that the level at which the response to the 500 Hz burst appeared was much more closely related to the amount of hearing loss at low frequencies than the loss at high frequencies. A good test is afforded by some of their patients, selected because they had their greatest hearing loss in the low-frequency region. For these patients, the basal end is presumably more sensitive to a 500 Hz signal than the apical end. If the response recorded is coming from the basal end, then adding a high-pass masking noise should change the level at which the effect appears and also change the latency. For the patients measured by Yamada *et al.*, those with low frequency losses showed no change in recorded FFR pattern when the high-pass noise was introduced. They feel they were measuring the response of the low-frequency end of the membrane. The simultaneous use of tone bursts and high-pass noise shows promise.

The use of short restricted-frequency signals should certainly be explored further in the audiology clinic. To establish that a young child has a hearing loss is useful, but to determine whether it covers the frequency range is even more useful.

Central Dysfunction 17

What is a central auditory dysfunction? Most experts would probably agree that if there is a malfunction of some part of the auditory system beyond the VIIIth nerve it might be useful to regard that as a central auditory disorder. What, then, are its manifestations? Conventional wisdom has it that one differentiating characteristic of central auditory disorders is normal or near normal sensitivity in the face of difficulty in understanding speech. This is not to say that sensitivity loss never accompanies central dysfunction, but rather that loss of sensitivity is attributed to peripheral disorder and central dysfunction usually occurs without any sensitivity loss. This makes it also somewhat clearer that central loss means, as we might expect, loss of some function or functions more complex than the response to simple tones. The assumption is that the processing of sound, in the sense of recognizing strings of speech sounds, classifying environmental sounds, etc., begins further up the brain stem than the VIIIth nerve.

Consequently one working rationale for assigning a "central" label to an auditory disorder is that it manifests itself *only* in the processing of such meaningful signals as speech or the sounds of other familiar sources. If the response to the various configurations of pure tones in the audiometry battery is essentially normal, the assumption is that only a central disorder exists.

But such considerations may be purely academic. The more practical question is: What is the role of the hearing specialist in malfunctions of the system central to the VIIIth nerve? Only rarely will the hearing symptoms be the first indication for the patient himself that something is amiss. Usually it will be some more general sign of illness that leads instead to the neurologist. Unless in the patient's reporting of his symptoms some special emphasis is placed on perception of speech or other sounds, the otologist or audiologist does not enter the picture. Brain scanning techniques are now so easily accomplished that non-invasive discovery of even fairly small tumors is the rule.

Some form of auditory test, then, for such patients would be sufficiently useful only if it can claim to detect or help to detect a tumor earlier, more conveniently or more safely than extant methods. If the auditory test is truly more convenient, or safer, the process can be fairly straightforward. With the tumor identified by the accepted method the patient is given the new test and the correspondence of the two procedures established. One now has a choice of either test, depending on preference or convenience. To establish that a new test leads to earlier detection is much more complicated. One must presumably use both procedures on suspected cases and establish that false negative cases by the old procedure that test positive with the new one become *bona fide* cases with the passage of time.

Following such a sequence for tumors beyond the level of VIIIth nerve obviously requires expertise both in neurology and in audition, plus access to suitable patients, along with some faith in the eventual worth of such tests. But even if we dismiss the diagnostic or discovery potential of auditory tests for central dysfunction, there is still good reason for the auditory expert to retain an interest in how auditory performance differs in the presence of central lesions. We know so little about how the auditory brain stem does its processing of complex signals that assessment of the changes in auditory perception once the location and extent of the lesion are verified can allow at least a glimpse of areas that are otherwise hidden from experimental view. Lesions in the brain stem and brain of experimental animals can tell us very little about the location of the functions performed in processing speech or music.

Tests with Speech Materials

The logical approach to an understanding of the relations between central lesions and specific auditory anomalies is to find the salient measurable ways in which persons with verified involvement of central auditory structures behave differently from those with normal central auditory systems. The modern era of this avenue of approach goes back to Bocca *et al.* in 1954. They noted the fact that up to that time neither tonal tests nor speech testing had shown that the hearing of patients with temporal lobe tumors differed from normal hearers. They introduced the concept of taking the redundancy out of the speech signal when using it as a test. In this particular instance they passed the speech test items (monosyllabic words) through a 500 Hz low-pass filter. They then plotted the percentage of words correctly heard as the level of this distorted signal was increased from threshold to some level well above. Since the signal was so severely filtered, the percent correct never rose to 100, but the important datum was the difference in performance at the two ears. In the patients with temporal lobe tumors the ear opposite the tumor performed significantly more poorly than the ipsilateral ear.

In the twenty-five or so years since the Bocca *et al.* work a number of similar procedures have been proposed. They may involve dichotic listening, like the Staggered Spondee test, which feeds one spondaic word into each ear, but offsets the two so that the first syllable of one coincides with the second syllable of the other. Example:

Left ear: play-pen
Right ear: cow-boy

A variety of such interaurally offset items is given to the patient in the Staggered Spondee Word (SSW) test. In some, different syllables combine into new words, as above. In some they do not. Responses from patients with central disorders are reported to differ from others in predictable patterns. (See Brunt, 1978, for a recent report.)

Another long-known behavior of the auditory system has been revived and refined as a possible test of central disorder. Fletcher described in 1929 an interesting method of demonstrating binaural summation of signals. If one puts a low-pass filtered band of speech into one ear and a high-pass band into the other ear, one ear might be receiving only frequencies lower than 1 kHz and the other only frequencies above 1 kHz. In such an instance either signal listened to alone will sound quite distorted. However, when both signals are present simultaneously, even though they are still only to separate ears, a clear undistorted speech impression will result. The demonstration can be carried even further by moving the low-pass point down and the high-pass point up until the signal in either ear by itself is completely unintelligible. Still, even with severe restriction in either ear, the two signals together—one in each ear—will be highly intelligible.

This kind of binaural summation has been tried in a number of forms as a test for integrity of central function. In one of the most sophisticated forms, Palva and Tokinen (1975) chose two narrow bands—about half an octave wide—and compared their summation in each ear separately with the summation in the two ears. Thus their test report is of the form

Right ear
  Sum _____ %
                       _____ % Binaural
Left ear   Sum
  Sum _____ %

where the monaural scores result from both of the filtered bands being fed to one ear, and the binaural score comes from having only one band in each ear. One should recall that usually patients who are being tested for central problems show normal sensitivity, so the setting of levels need seldom be a problem.

The claim of the authors, in a report of over 2000 cases, is that in central lesions the ear opposite the lesion will show a poorer score than the ipsilateral ear and the binaural score will also be poor.

Some additional similar schemes have been tried including dichotically competing sentences and interaurally switched speech. Varying degrees of success in relating results to verified lesions are reported. Unless the auditory expert is working closely with the neurologist and has the opportunity to check his results on a variety of patients, the guessing game becomes merely academic. Only a few combinations with the right mixture of expertise appear to be working on the problem, and progress has been slow.

Some promise for eventual assistance in the diagnosis of central disorders is offered by the evoked response techniques. We looked earlier at the time-locked responses that are recorded within a 10 msec period of the signal onset. There are two additional recordable sets of evoked response. One of these, known as the middle potentials, appears between about 15 and 50 msec after the acoustic signal onset and is presumed to be generated in the mid-brain and the cortex. It requires unusually expert technique to record these middle-potential signals properly, but some knowledge of their genesis is gradually building. Even the early components, which we have seen can be highly useful for threshold measurement, can also be analyzed for the integrity of the central part of the system. Picton *et al.* (1977) point out that the latency of wave V varies in a predictable manner in the presence of cerebellopontine angle tumors, in multiple sclerosis and in other vascular and neoplastic lesions that affect the auditory pathway. Selters and Brackman (1977) suggest a technique for camparing the latency of wave V when stimulating one ear with that when stimulating the other, noting that latency of wave V will be greater on the side of the tumor if that tumor is pressing on the VIIIth nerve.

Whether any of these techniques, now used tentatively or only as supplementary indications, will develop to the point of aiding substantially earlier diagnosis of auditory brain stem and cortical lesions only time will tell.

Hearing Aids 18

The normally-operating auditory system, as we have seen, performs over an impressively wide intensity and frequency range. Consequently, the sounds that we make and those we encounter and interpret from our environment represent a correspondingly large range of operation. When the system no longer performs normally, this impressively large array of incoming sounds may have to be modified in some predetermined way to compensate for the reduced capacity of a given patient.

The simplest instance is that in which some mechanical dysfunction has reduced auditory sensitivity. This would seem to be the natural case for a hearing aid, which in its basic form is a complete miniature sound system, consisting of a microphone, amplifier and earphone. In such a simple instance, this amplifying system moves the level of sounds up so that those that were too soft for the system are above the raised threshold. In the case of a simple mild conductive loss there should still be enough operating range left to accommodate the normal span of everyday sounds. As we saw in our discussion of such conductive losses, this may nowadays be repaired by an operation on the middle ear, and such a repair may obviate the need for purchasing and wearing an external device, suffering the inconvenience of regularly replacing its batteries, and keeping it in repair. However, if the repair is not completely satisfactory or an operation is impractical for other reasons, even a simple conductive loss may best be alleviated by a hearing aid. In such an instance, straightforward amplification of sound to bring the sounds of everyday conversational speech up by 25—30 dB is no problem for even very small hearing aids.

Such an aid may be built to fit completely into the external ear, continuous with the earmold that projects into the auditory canal. The pick-up microphone in this instance will be about at the plane of the outermost part of the pinna; the volume control is accessible in this same plane, as is the access to the battery compartment. The output transducer is molded into the plug that is custom fitted into the patient's ear and delivers sound quite directly into the approximately 2 cubic centimeter volume left in front of the eardrum. The aid may also be tailored to a small banana-shaped case that fits behind the pinna. In this model, the microphone opening is usually at the front, and the output sound is fed out a tube that inserts into the ear canal. This type may also be made with a button type receiver that clips to an ear mold filling the concha and projecting into the ear canal. This arrangement is apt to be preferred when a fairly high acoustic output is needed, *i.e.,* when the loss is fairly severe. Most of these aids can furnish some acoustic gain—meaning a higher level of output signal than input signal—over a frequency range of about 300 Hz to 3 kHz. If the patient's only problem is that some of the signals normally encountered are too faint for his poorly functioning system, such amplifying aids may be of considerable help.

It happens, however, that even for conductive losses, the loss is not the same at all frequencies. The usual configuration shows a progressively greater loss at higher frequency. What this probably implies is that whenever the mechanical transmission system is faulty in one or more of the ways listed in Chap. 12, even though the system becomes stiffer, the major effect is to require a greater mass (probably of bone) to be moved in transmitting vibration to the cochlea. Increasing the mass of a vibrating system lessens its response to higher frequencies.

For this and like reasons, one thing that may be done in a hearing aid in addition to straight amplification is some degree of tone control—frequently emphasizing the high frequencies as intimated. In addition to this kind of high frequency emphasis, it may be that low frequencies, to which this ear is more sensitive, and which tend to mask high frequencies, need to have less than average gain. So frequency equalization may be employed in the aid to make the gain at low frequencies close to one or even less than one.

Because hearing loss configurations can be very steep, as shown, for example, by the audiogram in Fig. 84, something more than frequency equalization may be required. What would probably be done here—depending on measures other than the audiogram—would be to pass through the hearing aid only frequencies from 1 kHz to 3 kHz or above. In other words, the gain at other frequencies would be much less than one. Even though this sharp restriction of the frequency range is called filtering rather than equalization, it is simply the same process to a greater degree. But band-pass filtering to present only part of the frequency range to ears with certain anomalies is another modification that can be accomplished readily in the modern electronic hearing aid. If the ear has near-normal sensitivity in some frequency range, the optimum amplification system may be one that leaves the ear canal open for reception of sound in that range and provides for leading in the amplified sound (in the defective range) by means of a small tubing that has little effect on the direct sound.

We noted in discussing cochlear disorders that frequently such a loss may mean that sounds grow rapidly in loudness and reach uncomfortable loudness not very far above the patient's (shifted) threshold. This situation creates a potential problem in the reception of the speech signal. Even for a constant level of speech production, the weakest sounds are almost 30 dB lower in level

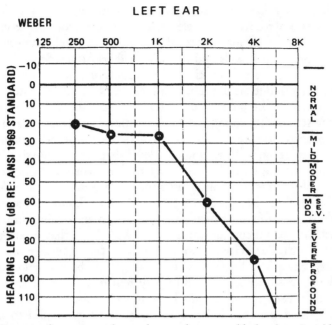

Fig. 84. Audiogram of a patient whose other ear has no usable hearing. An aid that passes only frequencies above 1 kHz might be of help. (See text)

than the strong sounds. In addition to this variation in the level of different speech sounds, the average level of speech production can vary 20 dB or more in different listening environments. If a listener's discomfort threshold for speech sounds is only 20 to 30 dB above his Speech Reception Threshold it is inevitable that many of the soft sounds of speech will be inaudible if the strong sounds of loud speech are kept at or just below discomfort level.

In theory, at least, this situation can be alleviated by wearing a hearing aid with provision for compression of the signal. This is done by having one stage of the hearing aid amplifier be a voltage-controlled amplifier. This is an amplifier whose gain is determined by the amount of voltage at one of its inputs. Then compression of the range of speech signals is accomplished quite simply electronically by using the signal waveform itself to create a voltage that is proportional to the average level of the signal. This is done by rectifying and partial smoothing of the speech signal. This relatively slowly varying voltage is then used to set the gain of the system so that—past a certain level, at least—the stronger the signal the lower the gain.

From the description above of the nature of the variation of level in speech sounds, it is apparent that two kinds of level compression might be useful for patients with a narrowed audible range. One would have the purpose of compensating for the variations in long-term average level, i.e., for the difference between loud speech, conversational and soft speech and the changes in level attendant on changes in distance between speaker and listener. Such a compression circuit is designed to react very slowly, meaning the rectified voltage has been smoothed until its variations take place in seconds.

Actually it usually has an onset time—attack time—of a few hundreds of milliseconds and a recovery, or release, time of the order of several seconds. This still leaves the normal range of variation in level between individual sounds like the strong vowels and the unvoiced fricatives. Smoothing out these variations requires the second kind of compression. In a compression device intended to smooth out the difference in level between strong and weak sounds, the difference is in the amount of smoothing applied to the rectified speech signal in the stage with voltage-controlled gain. At normal speaking rates the successive sounds of speech (phonemes) may be produced at an equivalent rate of 30 per second. Variations in level between successive sounds are minimized by cutting back the gain very rapidly when a strong sound comes along (control-voltage rise times of about a millisecond) and letting gain recover to normal at phonemic rates (30 to 40 msec). Unfortunately, even with modern electronics this is difficult to accomplish in a miniature amplifying system without introducing unwanted pops and thuds that interfere with the recepion of speech. Furthermore, we probably have to consider that smoothing out intensity variations between sounds may itself be distortion of the time pattern of speech so far as the auditory system is concerned. In this instance we have to discover whether it is the lesser of two evils.

Most of the experience in application of these principles to hearing aid wearers has been in formal experimentation and laboratory testing rather than in everyday normal hearing aid usage. There are commercial hearing aids with compression, but we have no good data on how successful it is. Experiments with various forms of compression have been pursued over the last 30 years. In 1952 Edgarth wrote about the possible advantages of compressing the dynamic range of speech sounds, but at that period it was technically difficult to do so. Even with modern improvements in compression techniques, demonstrations of the benefits of compressed speech have not been totally convincing. Comparisons have been made of the intelligibility, for hearing aid wearers, of compressed speech and speech that has had amplitude variation limited simply by clipping the high-amplitude peaks. Compressed speech has shown little or no advantage, though it sounds much better than clipped speech to the normal ear. Perhaps one reason for this limited success is the fact that compression has been applied to the total waveform of speech. One way the cochlea looks at speech is as a signal already separated into frequency bands. A better idea can be gained from Fig. 62, where it is apparent that for a steady level of speech reception the total range for any one set of receptors need not be so large as we may be led to believe when looking at the unfiltered speech waveform. The fact that amplitude compression for equalizing the levels of different speech sounds is a very difficult process without adding extraneous transients may mean that we have not aided speech processing very much, but have introduced some confusing elements. In spite of several admirable attempts to test compression we have few data to vouch for its efficacy, and this places it in the category of attractive ideas still to be explored.

The more conventional compression, with longer time constants, is in use in a number of hearing aids and can be very helpful. It is especially useful for loss cases that leave only a fairly narrow range between threshold and discomfort and also show susceptibility to further threshold shift (see Chap. 15). These cases, in fact, may pose an extremely difficult problem for the audiologist. Imagine a school-age child with a hearing loss of about 70 dB and evidence of recruitment. A loss of that degree is within the range of help from a hearing aid. In practice, an aid with a gain of about 50 dB will be prescribed. But this means that ambient levels, which normally measure 60 dB SPL or so in much of the school child's environment, are now 110 dB SPL. We should remember that in the absence of conductive loss the cochlea is subjected to the normal exposure occasioned by levels of 110 dB SPL. We must be aware also that we do not know whether the reason for this patient's loss is the same as for a loss from noise exposure, *i.e.*, whether additional exposure would add to his loss.

The audiologist may recommend a regimen for assessing whether the added noise exposure is contributing to threshold shift. The hearing aid is to be worn for a few weeks and a careful check made on Hearing Levels at the end of that period. This is followed by a week without the use of the aid. Hearing Levels are checked again to see if recovery of some temporary shift is evident. If it is, there is a real problem in choosing an appropriate compromise between exposure on the one hand and lack of help on the other. In such cases, ideally all necessary sounds should be just above the patient's threshold with none of them very far above, and this calls for compressing the range of useful signals into possibly a 10 dB amplitude window. There is no simple solution.

When a patient has a hearing loss in both ears, then the question arises whether to attempt to restore binaural hearing. We saw in Chap. 11 that there are some definite advantages to hearing with two ears. But we saw also that advantages beyond localization of sound are difficult to demonstrate objectively. In cases of hearing loss where two hearing aids may be required, considerable additional expense is entailed and the decision must be made on a very practical basis. Because characteristics of loss differ in many ways and so do the listening requirements of patients, depending as they do on personal habits and job requirements, the decision whether to use binaural aided hearing is made on a highly individual basis, frequently including a short trial wearing the aids before making the decision.

Even when listening is restricted to a single channel, as, for example, when only one ear is functioning, a small part of the usual binaural advantage can be realized by strategic microphone placement. One such arrangement is the technique called Controlateral Routing of Signal (CROS), in which the signal from a microphone at the bad ear is introduced into the good ear. The earphone for this signal is mounted above the good ear, usually in a spectacle bow, and led into the good ear without interfering with the unaided signal normally impinging on that ear. The CROS arrangement shows the greatest advantage over monaural listening when the "good" ear has normal or near normal hearing in the low frequencies but a loss in the highs. By the nature of the tubing arrangement that brings in the amplified (opposite side) signal high frequencies are emphasized, so they complement the good-ear signal. The major advantage, of course, is elimination of the effect of head shadow for signals on the bad side.

A similar technique can be used when the better ear has a moderate loss. In this case there is a microphone for each side and the signals are mixed and fed to a single transducer in a conventional earmold. This is referred to as a BICROS arrangement.

It is evident that the modern hearing aid offers a variety in the way of frequency range, amount of gain, total power output, spectrum shaping and dynamic control of gain. In general, the method for selecting the appropriate value of these parameters for a given individual starts with the shape of the audiogram. This will give an indication of the average gain required and also indicate whether extreme tone control settings or possibly filtering will be advisable. If other measures indicate abnormally rapid growth of loudness or lowered upper limit of comfortable listening, then some form of limiting of the amplitude range must be provided.

In most audiology clinics, and particularly in the United States, where a truly large number of aids is available, selection is narrowed by comparing speech reception through a number of suitable aids. This may be further supplemented by speech tests in interfering noise. More and more this use of interference in the clinic features some attempt at realism by using party noise or crowd noise, frequently over-dubbed repeatedly so that many statistical properties of interfering speech are preserved but the distraction of hearing the context of the interfering message is obviated.

The rationale for this comparison of aids through speech reception and speech against interference has been argued empirically rather than theoretically. The variability inherent in testing with monosyllabic word tests of a practical length is sufficiently large compared to differences between aids that the choice of one aid over another must be considered as heavily weighted with art as with measurement science. In spite of conscientious efforts by audiologists to improve these procedures, a recent report indicated one half the hearing aids purchased end up not being worn. It should be added that it is not known whether that proportion would change if all hearing aid purchasers availed themselves of audiology services.

The failure of non-conductive losses to respond more favorably to straight amplification or even selective amplification offers additional proof that cochlear and neural losses are not simply loss of sensitivity. One hopes that with increased knowledge of the function of the cochlea and the exact nature of auditory processing of speech the feasibility of remedial electronics will increase.

Auditory Implants 19

In certain cases of almost total deafness, the hair cells are non-functional but the VIIIth nerve is spared. In such instances the direct electrical stimulation of the nerve endings to restore some sensation of hearing has seemed worth investigating. No one entertains seriously the idea of duplicating the hair-cell-nerve interface by ascertaining how many effectively separate connections there are from hair cell to nerve. Not only would it be too difficult technically, but we do not know the number or precise nature of such connections.

Actually we are indulging in fantasy if we speak of imitating the cochlear connections to the nerve in detail. Current implants (1980) are a far cry from that pattern; and how much more sophistication they will attain depends heavily on greater promise of success.

There are, in general, three styles of electrical implant currently in operation. The simplest one feeds a single electrical signal to whatever nerves it activates. It may introduce the electric field with a single active electrode or with an array of electrodes, the latter intended to insure the stimulation of a greater spread of nerve fibers. The form of the electric signal may be simply the raw waveform like that of an amplified microphone signal, or it may be modified in ways that take some account of the limitations of feeding complex sound information directly to the nerves. These modifications may include compressing the amplitude range of the signal, using the electrical replica of the sound wave to modulate a suitable carrier or transposing and repacking the information into a frequency range better suited to the limitations of nerve fiber response. A number of patients have worn such devices for several years, and they do receive enough benefit to be convinced of the efficacy of wearing the device. Improvement in speech reception has not been demonstrable on objective testing, though most long-term wearers feel it takes place.

Limitations of the single-signal electric implant have led to the two other types, both of them featuring more than one information channel. This affords the opportunity to pre-code complex signals such as speech into a form that can be distributed over a small number of channels with not a very demanding requirement for high information capacity in any one channel.

The second of the three types of implant is accomplished by placing a small bundle of wires in the VIIIth nerve just central to the modiolus, as shown in Fig. 85. The wires are small in diameter (about 75 μ) and are insulated except at the tip. They are cut to different lengths so that the bare tip of each one is close to a different sample of nerve fibers. To the extent that these are independent samples, we have four different channels of information. In one scheme being tried (Simmons et al., 1979) each channel is fed some important attribute of the speech signal. For example, one channel might receive information on the movement of Formant I, the lowest resonance in the speech signal. Another channel can be fed with the analog of the move-

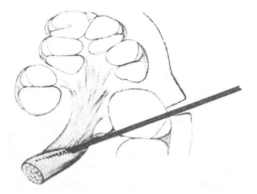

Fig. 85. The path of the electrode to the VIIIth nerve. The bundle of small wires goes through a hole drilled in the promontory (see Fig. 81), through the scala vestibuli and into the nerve as it passes through the temporal bone to the brain stem. (From Simmons et al., 1979)

ment of the second resonance, Formant II; and still another might be the presence or absence of fricative information, with another for intonation pattern or some other salient feature of the speech signal. All this information is distributed as nearly as possible, to the combination of electrodes that will maximize the similarity of the new sounds with the patient's former hearing. For example, the electrode with the lowest pitch (quality) of sound might carry intonation pattern, the next lowest first formant (low resonance) information, the next second formant (middle resonance) information, etc. Information is fed in at vibratory rates that are within the handling capacity of direct nerve stimulation. This scheme is just being introduced to patients and as yet has not shown the expected superiority over the single signal.

The third implanting scheme—the most appealing intuitively—places the wires directly into the cochlea, usually through the round window into the scala tympani as shown in Fig. 86. With careful placement of the electrodes, stimulation of a fairly small population of nerve fibers by each electrode is possible (Merzenich, 1979). Since the dendrites or cell bodies in and near the spinal ganglion are arrayed from the low to the high frequency end of the cochlea, the restricted sample under any given electrode in this

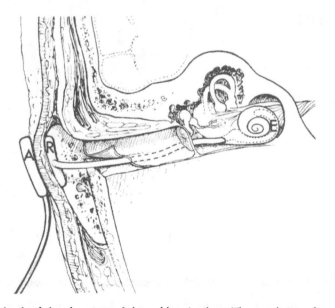

Fig. 86. A sketch of the placement of the cochlear implant. The speech (or other audio) signal is used to modulate a carrier and this is fed to the driving antenna coil *(A)*. This signal is picked up by the receiving coil *(R)*, demodulated and fed to the electrode *(E)* in the cochlea. (From Merzenich, 1975)

instance might be expected to have the sound of a narrow-band signal. It follows also that the sound of different electrodes would differ most from each other with such a system. Unfortunately, this pattern of stimulation, though it does seem to lead to a different quality of sound from each electrode position does not necessarily elicit a tone-like perception. Indeed there seems to be little universally reported resemblance between the new sounds and sounds previously experienced.

There are other problems with the attempt to restore hearing through electrical stimulation. The range between threshold and maximum tolerable level is relatively narrow—probably 12—15 dB at best— and we do not at this juncture know the number of dynamically differentiable steps in intensity. Pitch does vary with frequency of the applied signal, whether that signal is sinusoidal or a train of pulses, but only up to 500—700 Hz equivalent rate, and it also varies appreciably with changes in intensity.

No patients with sufficient training or experience with this third style of device have yet been reported. It is undoubtedly scheduled for a thorough evaluation over the next few years. The likelihood of more than marginal speech reception through this mechanism seems low, but for patients with no input through the acoustic channel, even the current stage of development offers enough help to recommend its use.

References

Anderson, C. M. B., Whittle, L. S. (1971): Physiological noise and the missing 6 dB. Acustica *24*, 261—272.

Anson, B. J., Donaldson, J. A. (1967): The Surgical Anatomy of the Temporal Bone and Ear. Philadelphia: W. B. Saunders.

Batteau, D. W. (1967): The role of the pinna in human localization. Proc. Royal Soc. (Lond.) *B 168*, 158—180.

Batteau, D. W. (1968): Listening with the Naked Ear. In: The Neuropsychology of Spatially Oriented Behavior (Freedman, S. J., ed.). Homewood, Ill.: The Dorsey Press.

Békésy, G. v. (1949): On the resonance curve and the decay period at various points on the cochlear partition. J. Acous. Soc. Am. *21*, 245—254.

Békésy, G. v. (1953): Shearing microphonics produced by vibrations near the inner and outer hair cells. J. Acous. Soc. Am. *25*, 786—790.

Békésy, G. v. (1960): Experiments in Hearing. New York: McGraw-Hill.

Bismarck, G. v. (1974): Timbre of steady sounds: A factorial investigation of its verbal attributes. Acustica *30*, 146—159.

Blodgett, H. C., Wilbanks, W. A., Jeffress, L. A. (1956): Effect of large interaural time differences on the judgment of sidedness. J. Acous. Soc. Am. *28*, 639—643.

Bocca, E., Calearo, C., Cassinari, V. (1954): A new method for testing hearing in temporal lobe tumors: Preliminary report. Acta Otolaryngol. *44*, 219—221.

Brunt, M. A. (1978): The Staggered Spondaic Word Test. In: Handbook of Clinical Audiology (Katz, J., ed.). Baltimore: Williams & Wilkins.

Butler, R. A. (1969): Monaural and binaural localization of noise bursts vertically in the median sagittal plane. J. Aud. Res. *3*, 230—235.

Buytendijk, F. J. J., Meesters, A. (1942): Duration and course of the auditory sensation. Commentationes Pontif. Acad. Sci. *6*, 557—576.

Campbell, R. A., Lasky, E. Z. (1967): Masker level and sinusoidal signal detection. J. Acous. Soc. Am. *42*, 972—976.

Cardozo, B. L. (1962): Frequency discrimination of the human ear. Paper H 16, Fourth International Congress on Acoustics.

Carhart, R., Porter, L. S. (1971): Audiometric configuration and prediction of threshold for Spondees. J. Sp. Hear. Res. *14*, 486—495.

Cherry, E. C., Taylor, W. K. (1954): Some further experiments on the recognition of speech with one and two ears. J. Acous. Soc. Am. *26*, 554—559.

Chih-an, L., Chistovich, L. A. (1960): Frequency difference limens as a function of tonal duration. Sov. Phys. Acoust. *6*, 75—80.

Chow, K. L. (1951): Numerical estimates of the auditory central nervous system of the rhesus monkey. J. Comp. Neurol. *95*, 159—175.

Corso, J. F., Levine, M. (1965): Pitch-discrimination at high frequencies by air- and bone-conduction. Am. J. Psychol. *78*, 557—566.

Davis, H. (1976): Principles of electric response audiometry. Ann. Otol. Rhinol. Lar. *85*, Suppl. 28.

Davis, H. (1978): Anatomy and Physiology of the Auditory System. In: Davis, H., Silverman, S. R.: Hearing and Deafness, 4th ed. New York: Holt, Rinehart and Winston.

Davis, H., Silverman, S. R. (1978): Hearing and Deafness, 4th ed. New York: Holt, Rinehart and Winston.

Davis, H., Silverman, S. R., McAuliffe, D. R. (1951): Some observations on pitch and frequency. J. Acous. Soc. Am. *23*, 40—42.

Davis, H., et al. (1953): Acoustic trauma in the guinea pig. J. Acous. Soc. Am. *25*, 1180 to 1189.

DeBoer, E. (1977): Pitch Theories Unified. In: Psychophysics and Physiology of Hearing (Evans, E. F., Wilson, J. R., eds). London: Academic Press.

Deutsch, L. (1972): The threshold of the stapedius reflex for pure tone and noise stimuli. Acta Otolaryngologica *74*, 248—251.

Divenyi, P. L., Hirsh, I. J. (1974): Identification of temporal order in three-tone sequences. J. Acous. Soc. Am. *56*, 144—151.

Doughty, J. M., Garner, W. R. (1947): Pitch characteristics of short tones. I. Two kinds of pitch threshold. J. Exp. Psych. *37*, 351—365.

Duifhuis, H. (1973): Consequences of peripheral frequency selectivity for nonsimultaneous masking. J. Acous. Soc. Am. *54*, 1471—1488.

Durlach, N. I., Colburn, H. S. (1978): Binaural Phenomena. In: Handbook of Perception, Vol. IV, Hearing (Carterette, E. C., Friedman, M. P., eds.). New York: Academic Press.

Edgardth, B. H. (1952): The use of extreme limitation for the dynamic equalization of vowels and consonants in hearing aids. Acta Otolaryngol. *40*, 376—382.

Efron, R. (1973): Conservation of temporal information by perceptual system. Perception Psychophys. *14*, 518—530.

Egan, J. P., Hake, H. W. (1950): On the masking pattern of a simple auditory stimulus. J. Acous. Soc. Am. *22*, 622—630.

Eldredge, D. H. (1974): Inner Ear—Cochlear Mechanics and Cochlear Potentials. In: Handbook of Sensory Physiology, Vol. 5, Pt. 1 (Keidel, W. D., Neff, W. D., eds.). Berlin-Heidelberg-New York: Springer.

Eldredge, D. H. (1978): Electrical Equivalents of the Békésy Traveling Wave in the Mammalian Cochlea. In: Evoked Electrical Activity in the Nervous System (Naunton, R., Fernandez, C., eds.). New York: Academic Press.

Elliott, L. L. (1962): Backward masking. J. Acous. Soc. Am. *34*, 1108—1115.

Elliot, L. L. (1971): Backward and forward masking. Audiology *10*, 65—76.

Evans, E. F. (1975): Cochlear Nerve and Cochlear Nucleus. In: Handbook of Sensory Physiology, Vol. 5, Pt. 2 (Keidel, W. D., Neff, W. D., eds.), Chap. 1. Berlin-Heidelberg-New York: Springer.

Evans, E. F. (1978): Peripheral Auditory Processing in Normal and Abnormal Ears. Scand. Audiol., Suppl. *6*, 10—47.

Evans, E. F., Wilson, J. P. (1973): The Frequency Selectivity of the Cochlea. In: Basic Mechanisms in Hearing (Møller, A., ed.). New York-London: Academic Press.

Flanagan, J. L., Guttman, N. (1960): On the pitch of periodic pulses. J. Acous. Soc. Am. *32*, 1308—1319.

Flanagan, J. L., Watson, B. J. (1966): Binaural unmasking of complex signals. J. Acous. Soc. Am. *40*, 456—468.

Fletcher, H. (1940): Auditory patterns. Rev. mod. Phys. *12*, 47—65.

Fletcher, H., Munson, W. A. (1933): Loudness, its definition, measurement and calculation. J. Acous. Soc. Am. *5*, 82—108.

Freedman, S. J., Fisher, H. G. (1968): The Role of the Pinna in Auditory Localization. In: The Neuropsychology of Spatially Oriented Behavior (Freedman, S. J., ed.). Homewood, Ill.: The Dorsey Press.

Gardner, M. B., Gardner, R. S. (1973): Problem of localization in the median plane: Effect of pinnae cavity occlusion. J. Acous. Soc. Am. *53*, 400—408.

Gescheider, G. (1966): Resolving of successive clicks by the ears and skin. J. Exp. Psychol. *71*, 378—381.

Ginsberg, I. A., White, T. P. (1978): Otological Considerations in Audiology. In: Handbook of Clinical Audiology (Katz, J., ed.). Baltimore: Williams & Wilkins.

Goldberg, J. M. (1975): Physiological Studies of Auditory Nuclei of the Pons. In: Handbook of Sensory Physiology, Vol. 5, Pt. 2 (Keidel, W. D., Neff, W. D., eds.), Chap. 2. Berlin-Heidelberg-New York: Springer.

Goldstein, J. L. (1973): An optimum processor theory for the central information of the pitch of complex tones. J. Acous. Soc. Am. *54*, 1496—1516.

Goldstein, M. H., Abeles, M. (1975): Single Unit Activity of the Auditory Cortex. In: Handbook of Sensory Physiology, Vol. 5, Pt. 2 (Keidel, W. D., Neff, W. D., eds.), Chap. 4. Berlin-Heidelberg-New York: Springer.

Greenwood, D. D. (1962): Approximate calculations of the dimensions of traveling wave envelopes in four species. J. Acous. Soc. Am. *34*, 1364—1369.

Grey, J. M. (1977): Multidimensional perceptual scaling of musical timbres. J. Acous. Soc. Am. *61*, 1270—1277.

Guttman, N., Julesz, B. (1963): Lower limits of auditory periodicity analysis. J. Acous. Soc. Am. *43*, 610.

Haas, H. (1951): Über den Einfluß eines Einfachechos auf die Hörsamkeit von Sprache. Acustica *1*, 49—52. [An English translation of the German dissertation that preceded this article was published in: Audio Eng. Soc. J. *20*, 146—159 (1972).]

Hall, J. L., Lummis, R. C. (1973): Thresholds for click pairs masked by band-stop noise. J. Acous. Soc. Am. *54*, 593—599.

Halverson, H. M. (1927): The upper limit of auditory localization. Am. J. Psychol. *38*, 97—106.

Harris, G. G. (1968): Brownian motion and the threshold of hearing. Int. Audiology *7*, 111—120.

Harris, J. D. (1963): Loudness discrimination. J. Sp. Hear. Dis. Monogr., Suppl. 11, 1—63.

Harris, J. D. (1974): The Electrophysiology and Layout of the Auditory Nervous System. New York: Bobbs-Merrill.

Hirsh, I. J. (1959): Auditory perception of temporal order. J. Acous. Soc. Am. *31*, 759—767.

Hirsh, I. J., Bilger, R. C. (1955): Auditory-threshold recovery after exposures to pure tones. J. Acous. Soc. Am. *27*, 1186—1194.

Houtgast, T. (1974): Lateral Suppression in Hearing. Doctoral Dissertation, Free University, Amsterdam.

Huggins, W. H. (1953): A Theory of Hearing. In: Communication Theory (Jackson, W., ed.). London: Butterworths.

Jenkins-Lee, J. E. (1971): Pitch perception for minimum tone bursts: Single periods. Unpublished Ph. D. Dissertation, Stanford University.

Jerger, J., Jerger, S. (1971): Diagnostic significance of PB word functions. Arch. Otolaryngol. *93*, 573—580.

Jerger, S., Jerger, J., Mauldin, L., Segal, P. (1974): Studies in impedance audiometry II: Children below six years. Arch. Otolaryngol. *99*, 1—9.

Jestead, W., Wier, C. C., Green, D. M. (1977): Intensity discrimination as a function of frequency and sensation level. J. Acous. Soc. Am. *61*, 169—177.

Johnson, D. L. (1973): Prediction of NIPTS Due to Continuous Noise Exposure. AMRL Report No. TR-73-91, Wright Patterson Air Force Base, Dayton, Ohio.

Kiang, N. Y. S. (1965): Discharge Patterns of Single Fibers in the Cat's Auditory Nerve. Cambridge, Mass.: MIT Press.

Kiang, N. Y. S., Moxon, E. C. (1974): Tails of tuning curves of auditory nerve fibers. J. Acous. Soc. Am. *55*, 622—630.

Kirikae, I. (1960): The Structure and Function of the Middle Ear. Tokyo: Miv. Tokyo Press.

Klumpp, R. G., Eady, H. R. (1956): Some measurements of interaural time difference thresholds. J. Acous. Soc. Am. *28*, 859—860.

Koenig, W. (1950): Subjective effects in binaural hearing. J. Acous. Soc. Am. *22*, 61—62.

Levitt, H. (1971): Transformed up-down methods in psychoacoustics. J. Acous. Soc. Am. 49, 467—477.

Levitt, H., Rabiner, L. R. (1967): Binaural release from masking for speech and gain in intelligibility. J. Acous. Soc. Am. 42, 601—608.

Licklider, J. C. R. (1951): Basic Correlates of the Auditory Stimulus. In: Handbook of Experimental Psychology (Stevens, S. S., ed.). New York: J. Wiley.

Lochner, J. P. A., Burger, J. F. (1958): The subjective masking of short-time delayed echoes by their primary sounds and their contribution to the intelligibility of speech. Acustica 8, 1—10.

Luce, R. D., Green, D. M. (1974): Neural coding and psychophysical discrimination data. J. Acous. Soc. Am. 56, 1554—1564.

Lüscher, E., Zwislocki, J. (1947): The decay of sensation and the remainder of adaptation after short pure-tone impulses on the ear. Acta Otolaryngol. 35, 428—445.

Masterton, B., Diamond, I. T. (1967): The medial superior olive and sound localization. Science 155, 1696—1697.

Masterton, B., Diamond, I. T., Ranizza, R. (1969): The evolution of human hearing. J. Acous. Soc. Am. 45, 966—985.

McGill, W. J., Goldberg, J. P. (1968): Pure-tone intensity discrimination and energy detection. J. Acous. Soc. Am. 44, 576—581.

McClellan, M. E., Small, A. M., jr. (1967): Pitch perception of pulse pairs with random repetition rate. J. Acous. Soc. Am. 41, 690—699.

Merzenich, M. M. (1975): Studies on Electrical Stimulation of the Auditory Nerve in Animals and Man; Cochlear Implants. In: Human Communication and Its Disorders (Tower, D. B., ed.). New York: Raven Press.

Merzenich, M. M., White, M., Vivion, M. C., Leake-Jones, P. A., Walsh, S. (1979): Some considerations of multichannel electrical stimulation of the auditory nerve in the profoundly deaf: Interfacing electrode arrays with the auditory nerve array. Acta Otolaryngol. 87, 196—203.

Michaels, R. M. (1957): Frequency DL's for narrow band of noise. J. Acous. Soc. Am. 29, 520—522.

Miller, G. A. (1947): Sensitivity to changes in the intensity of white noise and its relation to masking and loudness. J. Acous. Soc. Am. 19, 609—619.

Møller, A. (1963): Transfer function of the middle ear. J. Acous. Soc. Am. 35, 1526—1534.

Møller, A. (1974): The Acoustic Middle Ear Reflex. In: Handbook of Sensory Physiology, Vol. 5, Pt. 1 (Keidel, W. D., Neff, W. D., eds.). Berlin-Heidelberg-New York: Springer.

Møller, A. (1978): Coding of time-varying sounds in the cochlear nucleus. Audiology 17, 446 to 468.

Moore, B. C. J. (1973): Frequency difference limens for short-duration tones. J. Acous. Soc. Am. 54, 610—619.

Munson, W. A., Gardner, M. B. (1950): Loudness patterns—a new approach. J. Acous. Soc. Am. 22, 177—188.

Neff, W. D. (1975): Behavioral Studies of Auditory Discrimination. In: Handbook of Sensory Physiology, Vol. 5, Pt. 2 (Keidel, W. D., Neff, W. D., eds.). Berlin-Heidelberg-New York: Springer.

Nordmark, J. O. (1978): Frequency and Periodicity Analysis. In: Handbook of Perception, Vol. 4 (Carterette, E., Friedman, E. M., eds.). New York: Academic Press.

Northern, J. L., Downs, M. P., Rudmose, W., Glorig, A., Fletcher, J. L. (1972): Recommended high-frequency threshold levels (8,000—18,000 Hz). J. Acous. Soc. Am. 52, 585—595.

Owens, E. (1964): Tone decay in eighth nerve and cochlear lesions. J. Sp. Hear. Dis. 29, 14—22.

Palva, A., Tokinen, K. (1975): The role of the binaural test in filtered speech audiometry. Acta Otolaryngol. 79, 310—314.

Patterson, J. H., Green, D. M. (1970): Discrimination of transient signals having identical energy spectra. J. Acous. Soc. Am. 48, 894—905.

Patterson, R. D. (1976): Auditory filter shapes derived with noise stimuli. J. Acous. Soc. Am. 59, 640—654.

Patterson, R. D., Nimmo-Smith, F. (1980): Off-frequency listening and auditory-filter asymmetry. J. Acous. Soc. Am. *67*, 229—245.

Penner, J. J. (1977): Detection of temporal gaps in noise as a measure of the decay of auditory sensation. J. Acous. Soc. Am. *61*, 552—557.

Pfafflin, S. M., Mathews, M. V. (1966): Detection of auditory signals in reproducible noise. J. Acous. Soc. Am. *39*, 340—345.

Pfeiffer, R. R., Kim, D. O. (1975): Cochlear nerve fiber responses: Distribution along the cochlear partition. J. Acous. Soc. Am. *58*, 867—869.

Pickles, J. O. (1975): Normal critical bands in the cat. Acta Otolaryngol. *80*, 245—254.

Picton, T. W., Woods, D. L., Baribeau-Braun, J., Healey, T. M. G. (1977): Evoked potential audiometry. J. Otolaryngol. *6*, 90—119.

Plomp, R. (1964a): The ear as a frequency analyzer. J. Acous. Soc. Am. *36*, 1628—1636.

Plomp, R. (1964b): Rate of decay of auditory sensation. J. Acous. Soc. Am. *36*, 277—282.

Plomp, R. (1966): Experiments on Tone Perception. Soesterberg, Netherlands: Institute for Perception RVO-TNO.

Plomp, R. (1976): Aspects of Tone Sensation. New York: Academic Press.

Rabinowitz, W. M., Lim, J. C., Braida, L. D., Durlach, N. I. (1976): Intensity Perception. VI. Summary of recent data on deviations from Weber's law for 1000-Hz tone pulses. J. Acous. Soc. Am. *59*, 1506—1509.

Resnick, S. B., Feth, L. L. (1975): Discriminability of time-reversed click pairs: Intensity effects. J. Acous. Soc. Am. *57*, 1493—1499.

Rice, C. E., Schubert, E. D., West, R. A. (1969): On auditory sensitivity at high frequency. Psych. Record *19*, 611—615.

Riesz, R. R. (1928): Differential intensity sensitivity of the ear for pure tones. Phys. Rev. *31*, 867—875.

Ronken, D. A. (1970): Monaural detection of a phase difference between clicks. J. Acous. Soc. Am. *47*, 1091—1099.

Ronken, D. A. (1971): Some effects of bandwidth-duration constraints on frequency discrimination. J. Acous. Soc. Am. *49*, 1232—1242.

Rose, J. E., Hind, J. E., Anderson, D. J., Brugge, J. F. (1971): Some effects of stimulus intensity on response of auditory nerve fibers in the squirrel monkey. J. Neurophysiol. *34*, 685—699.

Rouiller, E., de Ribaupierre, Y., de Ribaupierre, F. (1979): Phase-locked responses to low frequency tones in the medial geniculate body. Hear. Res. *1*, 213—226.

Russell, I. J., Sellick, P. M. (1977): Tuning properties of cochlear hair cells. Nature *267*, 858—860.

Scharf, B. (1978): Loudness. In: Handbook of Perception, Vol. IV, Hearing (Carterette, E. C., Friedman, M. P., eds.). New York: Academic Press.

Schouten, J. F. (1940): The residue, a new component in subjective sound analysis. Proc. Kon. Ned. Akad. v. Wetensch. (Amsterdam) *43*, 356—365.

Schroeder, M. R. (1959): New results concerning monaural phase sensitivity. J. Acous. Soc. Am. *31*, 1579 (A).

Schubert, E. D. (1975): The Role of Auditory Processing in Language Perception. In: Reading, Perception and Language (Duane, D. D., Rawson, M. B., eds.). Baltimore: York Press.

Sekey, A. (1963): Short-term auditory frequency discrimination. J. Acous. Soc. Am. *35*, 682—690.

Selters, W. A., Bruckman, D. E. (1977): Acoustic tumor detection with brain stem electric response audiometry. Arch. Otolaryngol. *103*, 181—187.

Shaw, E. A. G. (1974): The External Ear. In: Handbook of Sensory Physiology, Vol. 5/1 (Keidel, W. D., Neff, W. D., eds.). Berlin-Heidelberg-New York: Springer.

Shower, E. G., Biddulph, R. (1931): Differential pitch sensitivity of the ear. J. Acous. Soc. Am. *3*, 275—287.

Siebert, W. M. (1962): Models for the dynamic behavior of the cochlear partition. M.I.T. Res. Lab. of Electronics Quarterly Progress Report, No. 64, 242—258.

Simmons, F. B. (1964): Variable nature of the middle ear muscle reflex. Int. Audiol. *3*, 136—146.

Simmons, F. B., Mathews, R. G., Walker, M. G., White, R. L. (1979): A functioning multi-channel auditory nerve stimulator. Acta Otolaryngol. *87*, 170—175.

Sivian, L. J., White, S. D. (1933): On minimum audible sound fields. J. Acous. Soc. Am. *4*, 288—321.

Skinner, P., Glattke, T. J. (1977): Electrophysiologic response audiometry: State of the art. J. Sp. Hear. Dis. *42*, 179—198.

Soderquist, D. R. (1970): Frequency analysis and the critical band. Psychon. Sci. *21*, 117—119.

Spoendlin, H. (1975): Neuroanatomical basis of cochlear coding mechanisms. Audiology *14*, 383—407.

Steele, C. R. (1974): Behavior of the basilar membrane with pure-tone excitation. J. Acous. Soc. Am. *55*, 148—162.

Stevens, S. S. (1961): Procedure for calculating loudness: Mark VI. J. Acous. Soc. Am. *33*, 1577—1585.

Stevens, S. S. (1972): Perceived level of noise by Mark VII and decibels (E). J. Acous. Soc. Am. *51*, 575—601.

Stevens, S. S., Davis, H. (1938): Hearing, Its Psychology and Physiology. New York: J. Wiley.

Stevens, S. S., Newman, E. B. (1936): The localization of actual sources of sound. Am. J. Psychol. *48*, 297—306.

Stevens, S. S., Volkmann, J. (1940): The relation of pitch to frequency: A revised scale. Am. J. Psychol. *53*, 329—353.

Stevens, S. S., Volkmann, J., Newman, E. B. (1937): A scale for the measurement of the psychological magnitude pitch. J. Acous. Soc. Am. *8*, 185—190.

Taylor, W., Pearson, J., Mair, A., Burns, W. (1965): Study of noise and hearing in jute weaving. J. Acous. Soc. Am. *38*, 113—120.

Terhardt, E. (1974): Pitch, consonance and harmony. J. Acous. Soc. Am. *55*, 1061—1069.

Thalmann, R. (1975): Biochemical Studies of the Auditory System. In: Human Communication and Its Disorders (Eagles, E., ed.), pp. 31—44. New York: Raven Press.

Tobias, J. V., Zerlin, S. (1959): Lateralization as a function of stimulus duration. J. Acous. Soc. Am. *31*, 1591—1594.

Tonndorf, J., Khanna, S. M. (1970): The role of the tympanic membrane in middle ear transmission. Ann. Otol. Rhinol. Laryngol. *79*, 743—753.

Tonndorf, J., Khanna, S. M. (1972): Tympanic-membrane vibrations in human cadaver ears studied by time-averaged holography. J. Acous. Soc. Am. *52*, 1221—1223.

Wallach, H., Newman, E. B., Rosenzweig, M. R. (1949): The precedence effect in sound localization. Am. J. Psych. *62*, 315—336.

Watson, C. S. (1963): Masking of tones for the cat. J. Acous. Soc. Am. *35*, 167—172.

Watson, C. S., Franks, J. R., Hood, D. C. (1972): Detection of tones in the absence of external masking noise. I. Effects of signal intensity and signal frequency. J. Acous. Soc. Am. *52*, 633—643.

Wegel, R. L., Lane, C. E. (1924): Auditory masking and the dynamics of the inner ear. Phys. Rev. *23*, 266—285.

Wever, E. G. (1971): The mechanics of hair cell stimulation. Ann. Otol. Rhinol. Laryngol. *80*, 786—805.

Whittle, L. S., Collins, S. J., Robinson, D. W. (1972): The audibility of low-frequency sounds. J. Sound Vib. *21*, 431—448.

Wier, C. C., Jestead, W., Green, D. M. (1977): Frequency discrimination as a function of frequency and sensation level. J. Acous. Soc. Am. *61*, 178—184.

Wightman, F. L. (1973a): Pitch and stimulus fine structure. J. Acous. Soc. Am. *54*, 397—406.

Wightman, F. L. (1973b): The transformation model of pitch. J. Acous. Soc. Am. *54*, 407—416.

Winckel, F. (1967): Music, Sound and Sensation, A Modern Exposition. New York: Dover Publications.

Woolsey, C. N. (1960): Organization of the Cortical Auditory System. In: Neural Mechanisms of the Auditory and Vestibular Systems (Rassmussen, G. L., Windle, W. F., eds.). Springfield, Ill.: Charles C Thomas.

Yamada, O., Kazuoki, K., Hink, R. F., Hitoshi, Y. (1978): Cochlear initiation site of the frequency-following response: A study of patients with sensorineural hearing loss. Audiology *17*, 489—499.

Yeowart, N. S., Bryan, M. E., Tempest, W. (1967): The monaural M.A.P. threshold of hearing at frequencies from 1.5 to 100 c/s. J. Sound Vib. 6, 335—342.

Yost, W. A., Wightman, F. L., Green, D. M. (1971): Lateralization of filtered clicks. J. Acous. Soc. Am. 50, 1526—1581.

Zwicker, E. (1976): Psychoacoustic equivalent of period histograms. J. Acous. Soc. Am. 59, 166—175.

Zwicker, E., Flottorp, G., Stevens, S. S. (1957): Critical bandwidth in loudness summation. J. Acous. Soc. Am. 29, 548—557.

Zwislocki, J. J. (1957): Some impedance measurements on normal and pathological ears. J. Acous. Soc. Am. 29, 1312—1317.

Zwislocki, J. J. (1963): An acoustic method for clinical examination of the ear. J. Sp. Hear. Res. 6, 303—314.

Zwislocki, J. J. (1975): The Role of the External and Middle Ear in Sound Transmission. In: Human Communication and Its Disorders (Eagles, E., ed.). New York: Raven Press.

Zwislocki, J. J., Kletsky, E. J. (1979): Tectorial membrane: A possible effect on frequency analysis in the cochlea. Science 204, 639—641.

Zwislocki, J., Pirodda, E. (1952): On the adaptation, fatigue and acoustic trauma of the ear. Experientia 8, 279—284.

Zwislocki, J., Sokolich, W. G. (1974): Neuro-Mechanical Frequency Analysis in the Cochlea. In: Facts and Models in Hearing (Zwicker, E., Terhardt, E., eds.). Berlin-Heidelberg-New York: Springer.

Subject Index

Absolute sensitivity 48
Acoustic reflex 146
   decay 147
Air-bone gap 135
Alternate binaural loudness balance 139
Artificial ear 122
Audiogram 124, 167
Auditory fatigue 148
Auricle 7, 8

Backward masking 80
Basilar membrane 17, 18, 20
Beats 58, 92
Békésy audiogram 135
   fixed frequency 137, 138
   pulsed tone 136
   Type II 137, 138
   Type III 146
Binaural masking level difference 112
Binaural summation test 163
Bone conduction 128
Brain stem 34

Cents, frequency 55
Characteristic frequency 28, 29, 35, 51, 79
Claudius' cells 20, 21
Cochlea 17
Cochlear microphonic 23, 27
Cochlear nucleus 33
Cocktail party effect 115
Complex tones 60
   composition 64, 87, 90
   pitch 60
Compliance 128
Compression in hearing aids 166
Concha 7
Cone of confusion, sound localization 105

Conversational speech 141
   area 123
Cortex 36
   hearing area 37
Corti, organ of 20
   arches of 20, 22, 25
Coupler 45, 122
Critical band 60, 63, 82, 94, 99, 120
Critical ratio 94
CROS 169

Damage risk 153
dBA scale 150
Deiters' cells 20, 21, 25
Difference frequency 59

Ear canal 7, 9
Ear drum 9, 11, 12, 130
   perforation 132
   thickened 131
Efferent fibers 26
Endolymph 20, 24
Energy integration 49
Envelope, traveling wave 19, 27, 28, 96
Equal-loudness contours 70
Eustachian tube 1, 129, 130, 157
Evoked response 157
   latency 159
   origin 157
Excitation pattern 96
   temporal 77

Formant 88
   in implant devices 172
Frequency-following response 160
Frequency jnd 53

Frequency response
    ear 9, 47
    filter 97
    neuron 29
Fusion 78, 82

Haas effect 78, 82
Habenula perforata 21
Hair cells 20, 21, 22, 24, 25, 32, 56
Harmonic partials 60, 90
Hearing Level 14
Helicotrema 18, 19
Helmholtz' theory 2
High frequency limit, for pitch 48
Impedance 127
Impulse response of pinna 107
Impulsive sounds 153
Inferior colliculus 35
Injury, blast 153
Intelligibility of speech 144
Intensity jnd 71
Interaural difference
    in intensity 103
    in path length 101, 102
    in time 101, 102
Intertone 58
Intervals, musical 54, 64
ISO reference levels 123

jnd
    frequency 53
    intensity 71, 140

Lateral lemniscus 35
Lateralization 103
Law of first wave front 110
Loudness Level 70, 71
Loudness scale 68

Masking 75, 91
    backward 81
    for audiometric testing 127
    residual 76
Maximum storage length 83
Medial geniculate 36
Mel scale 52
Middle ear 11
    cross section 131
    equivalent volume 131
    fluid 131
    muscles 15
    reflex 132, 141
Minimum audible field 44, 45, 122
Minimum audible pressure 44, 45, 122
    comparison with field 46
Minimum energy 43
Minimum interaural time difference 108

Minimum time interval 79
Missing fundamental 61
Mobility 128
    of drum 128

Neural response 21
    VIIIth nerve, fiber 29, 51, 79
Noise exposure 149
    3-dB rule 153
Noise levels 151

Octave 52
Olivary complex 35
Organ of Corti 20
Ossicular chain 13, 14, 15, 16
    discontinuity 130
    fixation 130
Oval window 18

Partials 60
    and musical intervals 64
    inharmonic, pitch of 63
Pascal 45
Perforation of drum 132
Perilymph 20, 23
Periodicity pitch 57, 59, 61
    vs place 62
Phase 90
Phase locking 35, 37, 55
Phon 71
Physiological noise 46
Pillars of Corti 22
Pinna 9
    role in sound localization 106, 108
Pitch 51
    high-frequency limit 48
    low-frequency limit 47
    non-musical 65
    of noise bands 66
    of short tones 56, 65
    scale 51
Place principle 28, 56
Precedence effect 110
Probe-tube measurement 45, 122
Pulsation threshold 96
Pulsed Békésy audiogram 136
Rate of decay 76
Reactance 128
Recruitment 140
Reissner's membrane 20, 21
Resonant frequency 85, 87, 88
Reticular membrane 22
Round window 12, 18, 20
Roughness 58

Scala media 17, 20
Scala vestibuli 17, 20
Scale tympani 17, 20
Semi-tone 52, 55
Sensation Level 68
Sensitivity 15, 23, 29, 43
Signal-to-noise ratio 67
SISI test 140
Sone 68
Sound Level Meter 150
Sound Pressure Level 44
  of speech 141, 142
Sound shadow 102, 170
Speech Detection Threshold 141
Speech discrimination 143, 144
Speech Reception Threshold 142
Speech sounds 141
  levels 123
Spiral ganglion 20, 25
Spondee word test 142, 144, 163
  staggered 162
Spontaneous rate 30, 31, 32
Stapedius 15, 16

Stapes 12, 13, 14
Stria vascularis 20, 24

Tectorial membrane 20, 22
Temporal acuity 79
Temporal integration 49
Temporal order 81, 83
Temporary threshold shift (TTS) 74
  from hearing aid 169
Tensor tympani 15
Threshold 121
Timbre 85, 88, 90
Time-frequency problem 50
Time-locked averaging 156
Tone-decay test 145
Traveling wave 18, 19, 27, 28
Tuning curve 29, 51
Tympanic membrane (see ear drum) 8, 11,
  12, 14

Weber fraction 53, 72, 73
Word discrimination "roll-over" 144, 145
Word Discrimination Test 143

Acknowledgements

The following figures were used from other works with permission granted by the publishers and/or authors, respectively.

Figs. 1 and 5 from Anson, B. J., Donaldson, J. A.: The Surgical Anatomy of the Temporal Bone and Ear. Philadelphia, Pa.: W. B. Saunders Company. 1967.

Figs. 3 (modified) and 22 from Shaw, E. A. G.: The External Ear. In: Handbook of Sensory Physiology, Vol. 5, Pt. 1 (Keidel, W. D., Neff, W. D., eds.). Berlin-Heidelberg-New York: Springer. 1974.

Fig. 4 from Stevens, S. S., Davis, H.: Hearing, Its Psychology and Physiology. New York: Copyright © 1938 by John Wiley & Sons, Inc.

Fig. 6 from Tonndorf, J., Khanna, S. M.: Ann. Otol. Rhinol. Laryngol. 79, 743—753 (1970).

Fig. 9 from Békésy, G. v.: J. Acous. Soc. Am. 21, 245—254 (1949).

Fig. 10 from Davis, H., et al.: J. Acous. Soc. Am. 25, 1180—1189 (1953).

Fig. 11 from Wever, E. G.: Ann. Otol. Rhinol. Laryngol. 80, 786—805 (1971).

Fig. 12 from Davis, H.: Anatomy and Physiology of the Auditory System. In: Davis, H., Silverman, S. R.: Hearing and Deafness, 4th ed. New York: Copyright 1947, © 1960, 1970 by Holt, Rinehart and Winston, Inc. Copyright © 1978 by Holt, Rinehart and Winston.

Fig. 13 from Spoendlin, H.: Audiology 14, 383—407 (1975).

Fig. 14 from Eldredge, D. H.: Inner Ear—Cochlear Mechanics and Cochlear Potentials. In: Handbook of Sensory Physiology, Vol. 5, Pt. 1 (Keidel, W. D., Neff, W. D., eds.). Berlin-Heidelberg-New York: Springer. 1974.

Fig. 15 from Pfeiffer, R. R., Kim, D. O.: J. Acous. Soc. Am. 58, 867—869 (1975).

Figs. 17 and 18 from Rose, J. E., Hind, J. E., Anderson, D. J., Brugge, J. F.: J. Neurophysiol. 34, 685—699 (1971).

Fig. 19 from Neff, W. D.: Behavioral Studies of Auditory Discrimination. In: Handbook of Sensory Physiology, Vol. 5, Pt. 2 (Keidel, W. D., Neff, W. D., eds.). Berlin-Heidelberg-New York: Springer. 1975.

Fig. 20 from Woolsey, C. N.: Organization of the Cortical Auditory System. In: Neural Mechanisms of the Auditory and Vestibular Systems (Rassmussen, G. L., Windle, W. F., eds.). 1960. Springfield, Ill.: Courtesy of Charles C Thomas, Publisher.

Figs. 21 and 43 from Licklider, J. C. R.: Basic Correlates of the Auditory Stimulus. In: Handbook of Experimental Psychology (Stevens, S. S., ed.). New York: Copyright © 1951 by John Wiley & Sons, Inc.

Fig. 23 from Kiang, N. Y. S., Moxon, E. C.: J. Acous. Soc. Am. 55, 622—630 (1974).

Fig. 24 from Stevens, S. S., Volkmann, J., Newman, E. B.: J. Acous. Soc. Am. 8, 185—190 (1937).

Fig. 25 from Shower, E. G., Biddulph, R.: J. Acous. Soc. Am. 3, 275—287 (1931).

Fig. 26 from Wier, C. C., Jestead, W., Green, D. M.: J. Acous. Soc. Am. 61, 178—184 (1977).

Fig. 28 from Plomp, R.: J. Acous. Soc. Am. 36, 1628—1636 (1964).

Fig. 30 from Flanagan, J. L., Guttman, N.: J. Acous. Soc. Am. 32, 1308—1319 (1960).

Fig. 32 from Ronken, D. A.: J. Acous. Soc. Am. 49, 1232—1242 (1971).

Fig. 33 from Scharf, B.: Loudness. In: Handbook of Perception, Vol. IV, Hearing (Carterette, E. C., Friedman, M. P., eds.). New York: Academic Press, Inc. 1978.

Fig. 34 from Fletcher, H., Munson, W. A.: J. Acous. Soc. Am. 5, 82—108 (1933).

Fig. 35 A from Riesz, R. R.: Phys. Rev. 31, 867—875 (1928).

Fig. 35 B from Jestead, W., Wier, C. C., Green, D. M.: J. Acous. Soc. Am. 61, 169—177 (1977).

Fig. 36 from Lüscher, E., Zwislocki, J.: Acta Otolaryngol. 35, 428—445 (1947).

Fig. 37 from Munson, W. A., Gardner, M. B.: J. Acous. Soc. Am. 22, 177—188 (1950).

Figs. 38 and 39 from Plomp, R.: J. Acous. Soc. Am. 36, 277—282 (1964).

Fig. 40 from Kiang, N. Y. S.: Discharge Patterns of Single Fibers in the Cat's Auditory Nerve. Cambridge, Mass.: The MIT Press. © 1965 by Massachusetts Institute of Technology.

Fig. 42 from Elliott, L. L.: J. Acous. Soc. Am. 34, 1108—1115 (1962).

Fig. 44 from Bismarck, G. v.: Acustica 30, 146—159 (1974).

Fig. 47 modified from Wegel, R. L., Lane, C. E.: Phys. Rev. 23, 266—285 (1924).

Fig. 48 from Egan, J. P., Hake, H. W.: J. Acous. Soc. Am. 22, 622—630 (1950).

Fig. 49 from Fletcher, H.: Rev. mod. Phys. 12, 47—65 (1940).

Fig. 51 from Houtgast, T.: Lateral Suppression in Hearing. Doctoral Dissertation, Free University, Amsterdam. 1974.

Fig. 52 modified from Patterson, R. D.: J. Acous. Soc. Am. 59, 640—654 (1976).

Figs. 54 and 55 from Durlach, N. I., Colburn, H. S.: Binaural Phenomena. In: Handbook of Perception, Vol. IV, Hearing (Carterette, E. C., Friedman, M. P., eds.). New York: Academic Press, Inc. 1978.

Fig. 59 from Batteau, D. W.: Listening with the Naked Ear. In: The Neuropsychology of Spatially Oriented Behavior (Freedman, S. J., ed.), p. 123. Homewood, Ill.: The Dorsey Press. © 1968 by The Dorsey Press.

Fig. 60 from Gardner, M. B., Gardner, R. S.: J. Acous. Soc. Am. 53, 400—408 (1973).

Fig. 61 from Wallach, H., Newman, E. B., Rosenzweig, M. R.: Am. J. Psych. 62, 315—336 (1949). Urbana, Ill.: The University of Illinois Press. © 1949, 1977 by the Board of Trustees of the University of Illinois.

Figs. 62 (modified), 67, and 74 from Davis, H., Silverman, S. R.: Hearing and Deafness, 4th ed. New York: Copyright 1947, © 1960, 1970 by Holt, Rinehart and Winston, Inc. Copyright © 1978 by Holt, Rinehart and Winston.

Fig. 77 (modified) from Hirsh, I. J., Bilger, R. C.: J. Acous. Soc. Am. 27, 1186—1194 (1955).

Fig. 78 from Taylor, W., Pearson, J., Mair, A., Burns, W.: J. Acous. Soc. Am. 38, 113—120 (1965).

Fig. 83 from Skinner, P., Glattke, T. J.: J. Sp. Hear. Dis. 42, 179—198 (1977).

Fig. 85 from Simmons, F. B., Mathews, R. G., Walker, M. G., White, R. L.: Acta Otolaryngol. 87, 170—175 (1979).

Fig. 86 from Merzenich, M. M.: Studies on Electrical Stimulation of the Auditory Nerve in Animals and Man; Cochlear Implants. In: Human Communication and Its Disorders (Tower, D. B., ed.). New York: Raven Press. 1975.

CPSIA information can be obtained
at www.ICGtesting.com
Printed in the USA
BVHW021654180723
667439BV00003B/49